To Jim,

Prose in exchange for poetry.

Affectionately,

Eva

Caring AND Curing

Caring

AND

Curing

COMMUNITY PARTICIPATION

IN HEALTH SERVICES

by Eva J. Salber, M.D.

PRODIST

NEW YORK   1975

First published in the United States by
PRODIST
a division of
Neale Watson Academic Publications, Inc.
156 Fifth Avenue, New York 10010

© Prodist 1975
First Edition 1975
(CIP Data on final page)
Illustrations by Ira Rosenfeld
Designed and manufactured
in the U.S.A.

This book is dedicated to the people of Bracken Field who taught me the meaning of community participation. I have changed their names along with the names of the Health Center, the Housing Project and the City. I have not, however, changed what they told me though of necessity I can share with others only fragments of our conversations. I thank them all, including those whose interviews I most reluctantly omitted, for the trust and affection they gave me.

Contents

Foreword

The truest social history of any era is not to be found in the places to which we might turn first: the newspaper headlines, the acts of legislatures, the reports of commissions, or the publications of scholars. It is, instead, written in the lives of people. And if—as I believe—the social order is the most powerful determinant of the health of a people, and if we can learn to focus broadly enough when we look, then in the life stories of people we can find not only the data of individual sickness and health, of personal and family history, or of idiosyncratic events and social circumstances. We can also see what the social order means—what life was like—for whole groups of people: what was good or bad, healthy or unhealthy, just or unjust, liberating or oppressive. And then we will know more certainly the things in the society we must struggle to change.

There was a time, a century or more ago, when physicians and other health workers knew this, when they recognized a responsibility even greater than that to the individual patient, and when some of them at least, fought as reformers and revolutionaries for change in societies that compelled large numbers of humans to go hungry, to live in slums, to sent their children off to factories and mills, to work in dangerous and inhuman environments, to suffer racial prejudice and oppression, and therefore to be sick.

But that interest and that professional responsibility were submerged and almost lost in the explosive growth of scientific and technical knowledge in medicine. Armed at last with real powers of diagnosis and treatment, physicians became the technicians of cure and palliation. "Cause" was something microbiological or biochemical, not something social. The individual patient was the only concern—and if "social factors" contributed to his illness, it was probably his fault, and he—not the society—that needed fixing. Health services moved into hospitals and away from people, and grew increasingly costly. If—like money, power and political strength they were maldistributed, and least available to those who needed them most, that was not our professional concern. Finally, in parallel with the views of technological elites in other fields, it seemed clear that the health care system should be managed and

controlled by health professionals, not by consumers. The role of
consumers—of "ordinary people," and particularly of the poor
and the ethnic minorities—was to come to us, the health professionals, in "our" society, in our settings, on our terms, and at
our price, and then to do as they were told.

In the 1960's in the United States, in the name of civil rights,
equity, and a war on poverty, a new effort began to modify—if not
transform—the social order. Some health professionals were part
of it. They believed that the health services should be moved back
to the communities where people lived—and needed them. They
believed that health professionals should be allied with health care
consumers, not just with other professionals. They believed that
new institutions, such as neighborhood health centers, should be
created—and that the people who used them should have an equal
share in their control with the health workers who staffed them.
Some even believed that these new institutions, and this new alliance, should be used to spearhead other kinds of change: in housing, employment, education, transportation and other aspects of
social policy.

Among the first of these new health professionals was Dr. Eva
Salber, and among the first of these new institutions was the Health
Center she directed in the Bracken Field public housing project on
the edge of a city's black ghetto.

If one works—as Eva Salber did for years—in this new alliance, three realizations are likely to emerge.

The first is that patients are not just patients; they are citizens,
with views and knowledge, experiences and skills of their own to
bring to the staffing and direction of their own human service institutions.

The second is that their life stories reflect strengths, sometimes almost incredible determination and ability to survive, and
not just the medical and social pathologies that health professionals
are so prone to see in others.

The third is that these lives, or fragments of life stories, reflect
something more than individual or family experience. In the pages
that follow, some families grow and others splinter; some children
succeed, others fail; a new job is found here, a chance is lost there.
But there are echoes of larger forces. Technological displacement,
hunger and unemployment in rural Alabama or Mississippi send

thousands of families north, poorly skilled or prepared for urban life in an indifferent society that offers little alternative, but filled with hope for survival and a better chance for the children. In the name of good basic housing, a society built high-rise ghettos. The war on poverty was designed to benefit its generals most, while the troops found themselves in new dead ends, subject to new kinds of ambush. Those stories are here too, for those perceptive enough to see them. In that sense, these are not just fragments of life stories. They are an agenda for continuing social struggle.

It is significant—and typical of the ethic that motivates the new health professional—that Eva Salber has not interviewed a sample of her consumer colleagues at Bracken Field as "cases" or "patients," nor has she neatly organized, summarized or interpreted what they have to say into a professional report. Instead, they talk for themselves, and that is entirely appropriate to a new alliance of health workers and deprived citizens who seek change. For that effort is our *work*—but it is their *lives*.

H. JACK GEIGER, M.D.

Stony Brook, New York
October, 1974

Introduction

Doctors are trained in clinical rather than social aspects of medicine. I believe, however, that it is impossible to plan and deliver good medical care without an awareness of the life styles of the people for whom this care is planned. An understanding of the weaknesses, strengths and coping mechanisms of a patient-population is as essential to adequate medical care as is excellent clinical training. Care is often provided by professionals whose backgrounds are very different from their patients. When this is the case, it is of even greater importance to learn in what respects a patient's life circumstances influence the seeking of care, presentation of symptoms, and acceptance of medical assessment and intervention.

Health services will prove satisfactory only when patients and health professionals cooperate and collaborate, not only in the delivery of actual medical services, but also in an attempt to identify and solve community problems. In this partnership patients get better medical care. They also develop self assurance and recognize their potential power as a pressure group. At the same time, doctors who truly listen to their patients become more skilled physicians as they gain greater knowledge of human needs.

The interviews which follow are intended to illustrate these three main points. First, when patients and doctors collaborate in planning and delivering health services, the quality of those services is improved. Second, this collaboration benefits the patient not only medically but psychologically and socially as well. Third, the partnership between doctor and patient helps the doctor by giving him more profound understanding of the causation of illness and of its effects on the community.

The interviews which make up this book result from my experience in East City as Director of the Bracken Field Health Center located in a low-income housing project. The burdens of being both poor and black are discussed with bitterness, and at some length, by many of the people I interviewed. This was inevitable since the population of the project was mostly black. The concepts I have outlined, however, apply equally well to any population group. The Health Center and the interviews can be more fully understood if I provide some background material.

During the days of Johnson's "Great Society", many programs were funded by the federal government, mainly through the Office of Economic Opportunity, for the purpose of abating poverty. Some of these programs, and those of other governmental agencies such as the Children's Bureau, focused on populations with special health needs (high risk populations), such as the poor, certain groups of pregnant women, young infants.

For example, in 1965 the Office of Economic Opportunity funded the first Neighborhood Health Center in the United States. Each health center was to be responsible for the primary health care of a defined population whose income fell below a stated poverty level. The care was designed to be ambulatory, comprehensive in scope, continuous in nature and delivered with due regard for an individual's dignity. Furthermore, there was to be "maximum feasible participation" of the community to be served in the planning and governance of the center. Another prominent feature of policy design was the employment of as many community residents as possible to staff the health center.

The Maternal and Infant Care Program and the Children and Youth Program of the Children's Bureau, launched also in the 1960's, emphasized quality care to individuals at high risk of illness. The Maternal and Infant Care Program was designed to lessen the incidence of mental retardation in children by reducing premature births which, in turn, would be reduced by the provision of good prenatal and obstetric services to mothers. The Children and Youth Program provided quality care to children up to age 21. The Bracken Field Health Center was funded by grants from both these Children's Bureau programs.

The grants were received by two university teaching hospitals, one a maternity hospital, the other a children's hospital. I directed both programs as a single combined program. The future site for the operation of these programs had been chosen before I became Director—it was to be located in a low-income housing project situated approximately one mile from the two hospitals. The choice of location stemmed from the existence on this site of an unusual university-based mother and child health program. The population group I served had also already been selected. It consisted of mothers and children living in the housing project itself, Bracken Field, and those who lived in a defined geographic area surrounding the project in a section of the city named West Hill. Though eligibility was restricted initially to mothers and children, I was determined that one day the clinic would become a neighborhood health center serving all family members. I was eager to foster the consumer viewpoint, eager to employ community residents, eager to get to know the community.

The compelling reasons for the employment of community residents as staff members of a health center in the United States are well known: the scarcity of health manpower, the expense of using highly trained professionals for jobs which can be done by others less specialized, the psychological and cultural acceptability of neighborhood people, the role of the community resident as intelligent informant and bridge between health center professional staff and patients. The role of the community resident as exemplar is less obvious but equally important. Children of the ghetto tend from their earliest years to see themselves as failures. This image is counteracted as increasing numbers of individuals from minority groups fill positions of importance. In addition, community resident employees help to balance the usually overpowering dominance of professionals in setting policy by bringing to light the viewpoint of the consumers. We took over the existing dedicated staff of the mother and child clinic, including a few part-time community residents, renamed the clinic, and began planning the Health Center program in April 1967. Implementation of the program began in August of that year.

Bracken Field is like most low-income housing projects in East City. Though presumably built for the benefit of the poor, the entire project shows little planning with regard to the social amenities necessary for well-being. Buildings of red brick surround open court-yards of asphalt and concrete where few trees grow. These trees are protected from the children by iron palings. Laundry is strung up on lines adjoining the parking lots. The project is large, more than a thousand units, and is located within a residential section of East City. It is near a main shopping street, public transportation, schools, churches and hospitals. Within the project area itself, however, there are no supermarkets, small shops or laundromats. Besides a neighborhood house and a hall for meetings, there are no recreational facilities. There is a tot lot for small children provided with the usual playground equipment, but its concrete base is always strewn with broken bottles and rusted cans. Incinerators, inadequate for their loads, spill over with garbage. Piles of garbage are dumped by tenant children in hallways and gutters where rats and roaches multiply. Broken windows, or windows boarded up after fires, are a common sight. Maintenance and repair service is slow and inefficient. Hallways and stairs are dark and littered, most light bulbs are missing, graffiti are commonplace. Tenants avoid the elevators in the seven-story buildings, for fear of being trapped by a mechanical failure or in terror of being assaulted. But walking up six flights of unlit stairs is frightening, too. Apartments are numbered but have no bells, knockers or peepholes. Mailboxes, located in the vestibule on the ground floor, are frequently smashed and their contents pilfered, especially on the first and fifteenth days of the month, when welfare checks are delivered.

The manager of Bracken Field and his staff, whose office is within the project, deal with rentals, maintenance, evictions and complaints, but policy is controlled "downtown" by the East City Housing Authority. Until very recently, managers have been white, and none has ever lived within the project. Rents are on a sliding scale according to income. When the project was new, the tenant population was predominantly white, and occupancy was often gained through the influence of local government officials. Over the years there has been a steady exodus of white tenants, and the project has become 80 percent black. Entry for black tenants tends to be by way of social agencies rather than legislators.

Only the poor are eligible for low-rent housing, consequently almost all families who live in the project have problems. If there are husbands, they are often sick or disabled; most of the household heads are women with children to support. The children—an average of three per family—attend overcrowded schools, are behind in reading levels or drop out of school. Ill health, unemployment or low salaried unskilled jobs, inadequate police protection, exposure to criminal violence and drug abuse prevail. These citizens have only a small voice in matters affecting control of their lives. One section of the housing project is set aside for the elderly of whom almost all are white. These old people live as if imprisoned, afraid to leave their apartments because of the ever-present danger of purse-snatching and mugging.

Bracken Field, primarily a black pocket encased by a large

area called West Hill, a poor and lower middle-income white neighborhood, meets enmity and deep prejudice outside its boundaries. The inhabitants of the periphery are predominantly Catholic of Irish descent, although there is a steady influx of Spanish-speaking people to the area from Cuba, Puerto Rico and Central America. While those who live outside the project despise and fear those who live within it, they are not united themselves. Certainly the possession of a common language does not ensure unity.

My first six months as Director was devoted to recruitment and training of staff and to planning the delivery of services I hoped we would give. Since I knew that rational planning of services was not possible without at least a minimum of knowledge of the population structure in our designated area, the first two months were devoted largely to conducting a door-to-door population census.

We found, after preliminary analysis of these census data, that we would serve a little over 2,000 households containing 8,000 potential clients, mostly children. We knew also that when funding restrictions were removed, and we could serve all adults, our client population would approximate 17,000 persons. One third of the "eligible" households containing forty percent of the area's children were situated in the housing project, and sixty percent of those families depended on welfare payments for support. The majority of these households were black, and family units were often incomplete—without a father living in the home.

My plan was to divide the total area, initially, into two subareas, each to be served by its own health team, thus making it easier for patients and staff to get to know each other. Patients would be introduced to a team, rather than to an individual doctor, not only to permit the doctor more time for specifically medical problems, but also because other members of the team, themselves often from the community, might be more able to deal with a particular family problem. Each health team consisted of pediatricians, public health nurses, social workers and "neighborhood aides." The aides combined the functions of reaching out to residents of the area to invite them to come for services, with assisting nurses in the clinic and the field. They followed up on patients who had broken appointments, and assumed duties related to easing the way for patients to receive care. The nutritionist, the community psychiatrist, the obstetricians and the dental unit served both teams.

Patients were registered at the Health Center, given an iden- tification card and invited to make appointments for a complete physical examination. Patients were also seen without appoint- ments for examination and treatment if they spontaneously sought our care. When patients were admitted to hospitals they were vis- ited by Center staff members, and contact was maintained on dis- charge from the hospital. Since we focused on the family rather than the individual as the unit of care, mothers were invited to bring in the rest of the family when one member was registered or received care. We kept records of each family member within a family folder in which additional data pertinent to the entire family were recorded.

In the first year of our service we recruited fifteen percent of our staff from the area we served. By the end of the second year we recruited from the area more than one third of the staff of eighty persons. Community residents filled almost all clerical, secretarial, administrative and patient-care positions just below the pro- fessional level. We devised our own training programs, set up com- mittees to work on renovations, record keeping, clinic procedures, reporting mechanisms . . . and in six months we were ready for ac- tion.

We did not lack for patients. Twelve hundred families re- gistered with the Health Center during our first year of operation, and registration was heaviest among those families whose need for services was greatest—families with the lowest income, those who lived in the housing project, those with very young children, those receiving Aid for Dependent Children. Use of the Center's services by these registered families was heavy, and, again, those whom we judged to need services most used the services most often.

A small research unit under my direction monitored and evaluated the impact of our health services. We found utilization of services was even greater than anticipated. Mothers expressed satisfaction with the convenience of the Center, its friendly at- mosphere, the quality of medical care provided and the amount of time the doctors devoted to their care. Those mothers who had re- gistered were prepared to talk to doctors about emotional and behavioral problems; mothers who were not registered did not mention such problems. Exposure to our doctors gave mothers a different concept of the doctor's role than any they had held previously.

Let me return briefly to the period before services began and to the subject of consumer participation. While we were collecting and analyzing census data, planning patient services, and instituting staff in-service training programs, I was beginning to involve community residents themselves in all these activities. Our agency had been given a seat on the local Antipoverty Board. By becoming the agency representative, I was able to meet local opinion leaders and learn about community problems and strengths first hand. When sub-committees of the Antipoverty Board were formed I volunteered to be the chairman of their health committee. Two or three other board members joined that committee. This was the beginning of the Advisory Health Committee of the Bracken Field Health Center.

Our census takers had identified a few women who might be interested in joining our Health Committee and I urged all Health Center staff to encourage patients and potential patients to join. When it became obvious that we needed a full-time person to organize the kind of group and program I had in mind, an experienced community organizer was hired for the job. Together we recruited about twenty people who were willing to serve on the Advisory Health Committee. Eight of this group were interested enough to want to hold meetings twice a week in the initial stages. Most of the original eight lived in the housing project and remained stable members of the committee. About fifteen months after the Committee was initiated, and after repeated urging on my part, the group formed its own executive committee and I stepped down as chairman. They hired their own community advocate (paid by the Health Center) and became an incorporated body. Since all the Committee members were registered at the Health Center and most lived in the housing project, we got instant reactions to unmet needs and deficiencies in the services we provided.

As Committee members' knowledge, interest and confidence grew, they were drawn increasingly into the planning and operation of the Center. They were consulted on hiring and firing of key personnel, and on the disposition of the Center's budget. They met and discussed programs with each department head, and together with the Administrator of the Center, Committee members worked out grievance procedures for community residents and community staff to follow. All research involving the community that we or others proposed was discussed with the Committee, as it was with Center staff, and staff and Committee members received copies of research findings. To me these discussions and "feedback" were both a right and an educational tool to improve awareness of health problems and to devise better systems of medical care.

There were, inevitably, times when the Committee members overstepped their boundaries and interfered with the technical aspects of medical care, and relationships with Center staff were often ambivalent and even stormy. As the members' confidence grew, so did their demands for more share in decision-making. There was great need for patience, understanding, tolerance and education on both sides.

Shortly before I left the Health Center, we succeeded in establishing joint policy meetings between the eight community women, representatives of the university, directors of the two hospitals responsible for the program, and the chairman of the West Hill Antipoverty Program. Though these joint meetings were discontinued after I left the Health Center, the Health Committee remained an active force influencing planning and programs.

At the end of 18 months as director of the Bracken Field Health Center I resigned in protest over what I felt was a large, unwarranted budget cut imposed on us without any prior discussion or warning. Although I was angered and frustrated by the lack of a guaranteed long-term commitment that I and the community expected, and saddened by what I felt to be inadequate support in this crisis by those who had hired me, I stayed on an additional year until a new director was appointed.

There has been much criticism of the role of consumers in neighborhood health centers. While this book perhaps dwells more on the benefit to the individual than to the institution, I believe the benefit to both was clearly shown in the loyal support of the community in attempting to restore budget cuts, the pride and identification of the community in its health center, and the residents' desire to expand the boundaries of the center.

Aside from their primary and obvious purpose to provide medical care, health centers can serve as potential agents for social change in the communities they serve. I believe an active participation in community affairs can be invaluable to individual growth and to the individual's understanding of active citizenship. Participants in community affairs begin to believe that they have something to offer a society which has largely ignored them in the past.

There were several community members whose lives were radically changed during their years of participation in community affairs. Mark Clay, for some years a laborer, was appointed Director of Community Relations in East City Children's Hospital, became President of East City Antipoverty Board and was appointed to two Mayoral Commissions. Robert Prescott rose from laborer to Housing Manager of Bracken Field, and became an adviser on the Governor's Educational Committee. Frances Mitchell was appointed to the Board of an old and prestigious hospital; Celia Holder, Stella Jones and Nancy Early hold seats on every consumer organization in East City. Celia has become a community organizer for another health center, has bought her own house, and is well known in health circles far beyond the borders of East City. Many of those interviewed are taking educational courses in fields ranging from business to social anthropology. Sister Patricia, no longer on the staff of the Health Center, is a guidance counsellor in an adult education program housed in the Health Center complex. This program is preparing forty-five adult students for the high school equivalency examination and uses Health Center personnel in addition to regular teachers.

Important as these examples are, they perhaps are insufficient to show what at first I thought would be revealed through the interviews alone, without added interpretation. I wanted to make clear that good medical care cannot be separated from care of other human needs. Treatment of episodic illness, per se, does not improve the health of a community, though every individual wants and is entitled to relief from discomfort when ill. While this statement is true for any community, rich or poor, it is especially applicable to communities such as Bracken Field, where so much illness is social in origin and results from being poor in a culture which tends to associate poverty with shame.

This concept is difficult to get across even to health professionals, who have been educated and indoctrinated by specialists, in institutions designed to treat illnesses, often exotic illnesses, rather than people. It is little wonder that the gap between health professionals and the people they attend is wide. At the same time poor people, like everyone else, cannot minister to their own ills and need the technical skills of the professionals. An accommodation must be sought between the intellectualism and arrogance of many professionals, on the one hand, and the suspicion and hostility of many patients on the other. Such an accommodation is possible if professionals become willing pupils as well as teachers. If they can go far enough beyond medical care to join in their patient's struggle for better jobs, housing, education, security and recreation they will help to achieve better health for those they serve by improving the quality of life in a community. But joining the struggle is often a difficult, exhausting experience with few measurable rewards except the personal satisfaction of working with a small group of individuals towards a common goal.

Persons in positions of affluence and influence often say that the kind of people who speak through this book are shiftless, incompetent and unable to grasp abstract concepts or plan for the future. On the other hand, there is a tendency in some circles to imbue "community people" with almost magical powers in the belief that community control can solve a wide range of problems that a more traditional, established approach has failed to solve. Under-expectation and over-expectation are equally false. Both lead to mistrust, disillusion and frustration.

It is clearly unrealistic to expect that the mere act of forming a consumer committee, whether advisory or policy making, is sufficient to ensure participation in policy decisions. There is not only a large body of factual information about health services systems, and about local, state and federal resources that has to be learned, but beyond this consumers have to be coached, coaxed and encouraged to share their ideas with professional staff without fear of embarrassment or intimidation. Consumers cannot play a vital role in health center affairs without a properly organized and continuing program of education. Courses can be set up by health center staff, but it is preferable that such courses be offered by an outside agency in order to lessen any possible conflict of interest. Almost from the inception of the Advisory Committee we conducted our own training program but arranged for additional help from the East City Antipoverty Office.

Our training program covered other areas in addition to health and included such topics as governmental structure and financing, formation and functions of committees, structure of health delivery systems, composition of budgets, and specific role functions of Health Center personnel. Field trips were arranged to other health and community facilities.

With staff encouragement two additional health center-initiated committees were subsequently formed. One was the West Hill Health Committee which aimed at extending the Health Center to embrace all citizens of West Hill. This committee was successful in setting up a satellite clinic affiliated with the Bracken Field Center. The other was a Drug Committee set up because the constant theft of the Center's typewriters and adding machines by adolescents who needed cash to support their drug habits pointed to an urgently needed service.

There were other community organizations besides those connected with the Health Center. The West Hill Community Action Program, an offshoot of the East City Antipoverty Program, was well entrenched before the establishment of our Health Center, and was the most potent community organization in the area. Members of this organization over the years formed additional committees. One group took over the management of the Neighborhood House Community Center, another became a Tenant Management Committee which aimed at training tenants to maintain the Project on behalf of the Housing Authority. None of these committees was large and many had overlapping leadership. All struggled with inadequate budgets obtained through federal or local agencies, and they survived largely because of the energies of community leaders. I myself attended Bracken Field Health Advisory meetings, West Hill Health Advisory meetings, Community Action meetings, Drug Committee meetings and Crisis meetings, called whenever a critical incident occurred—children bitten by rats, a bomb threat, budget crises . . . .

When I left the Health Center in August, 1969 I joined another branch of the university in order to analyze data and write a series of quantitative reports on the services I had helped to establish. But the medical care needs of an impoverished population cannot be expressed adequately through tables and charts alone. As an adjunct to the analyses, therefore, I recorded interviews with people who worked or lived in Bracken Field—members of the Advisory Health Committee, members of other community organizations, Health Center employees. . . . During the interview sessions, I became completely involved in the narratives; they told of lives so poignant and rich in experience that I wondered whether the narrators might speak, with me, for the needs and desires of the community we represented. This idea became so increasingly compelling that when my husband accepted a new position in North Carolina, and we moved house in August 1970, I decided to take a sabbatical in order to present this book. 1974 finds me still working on the book, for I was drawn again to help organize a new neighborhood health center and later joined a university department leaving little time for writing. I feel, however, that what I and my interviewees have to say is important enough to persevere in the effort.

No interview took less than forty-five minutes; most lasted for at least one and a half hours, and several for much longer than that. I have more than eight hundred pages of single spaced typescript, unstructured except for my questions, often rambling and repetitious, but voicing tragedy, passion, love and hate and a longing to be recognized and heard.

How was I to share with others this outburst of feeling, this emotional expression, and make it readable, meaningful? It has been extraordinarily difficult for me to slash drastically and omit some interviews altogether in my final decision to highlight only three aspects of importance. The first is the contribution of community participation in medical services to the quality of that medical care. The second is the value of this involvement to the individuals who are involved. And the third is my equally strong belief that medical care cannot be divorced from a caring concern with other human needs if we as health professionals are sincere in our desire to help all communities attain better health.

Chapter I

Advisory Health Committee

Frances Mitchell — A Seeker of Knowledge

Frances Mitchell's outstanding quality was her equanimity. One of six children, she was born and brought up in East City. Though she herself had six children, between pregnancies she attended night school, determined to finish high school. She was both a stimulating and a calming force at meetings of the Advisory Health Committee and her influence (as the newspaper excerpt below reveals) was appreciated beyond the confines of the housing project.

Excerpt from East City Newspaper, May, 1971: East Huntington Hospital officials yesterday elected three neighborhood representatives to serve on the corporation and the board of trustees. The election marked the first time community people have been elected as trustees and the move marks the increasing interest of the hospital in neighborhood medicine. Elected to serve are . . . and Mrs. Frances Mitchell of West Hill . . . "

I really wasn't interested in organizations at all till I joined the Health Committee. When I first joined there were only three others already on the Committee, and at that time staff people were always at the meetings. There were so many staff it was funny. And the four of us community people were sitting there kind of nodding our heads like we really knew what was going on.

At first I had a hard time making the meetings because my friend went to work at the Health Center, and I took care of her three children. At that time I had six of my own and my sister's little boy; so I had ten children to look after. I used to come to meetings with some of the children, though I don't think I ever came with all 10 of them. When some of the children started going to school and I was back just to my own six again, I attended the meetings and found that, though I thought I didn't know what was going on, I had been learning all along. I don't know how much I've applied, but I can see that it's just been a fabulous experience.

For one thing, being on the committee helped me to become more aware of what is going on in the whole world. Not just the project I lived in, not just the Health Center and the people I dealt with in there, but it just opened up a whole new world of things. Health broadened into housing and schooling and even politics. We got a whole new learning of what was going on, especially when that budget cut came along. You know, we all started writing to our

senators and representatives and started seeing people on high
levels; I learned so much about how things are run and who is doing
what for us or who is supposed to be doing what.

You know how it is, being a mother your whole world is your
children; before that my whole world was social and fun. Who
cares . . . this happened . . . that happened. I couldn't get interested in things but I would try to read. But being involved and
really active with the Health Committee, I really began to know
what was going on, really began to have an opinion of things. I've
just gotten so stirred up the last couple of years that if I dropped out
of the Bracken Field Health Committee I'd have to get involved
with something else. Now that we are seeing some of the things we
dreamed of come about, we know they happen because so many
people put in so much time, so much effort, so much concern.

One of the things I got interested in through the Health Committee was the Tenant Management Committee. You know there's
a training program for the people on that committee. Even if the
idea fails and the money goes back to Housing and Urban Development I don't think it really would be a failure. We would have
learned so much about housing and so much about ourselves,
too,—how to structure, to try and get things going. If you fail in one
step, that gives you experience when you're onto something else.
We learn from each other too, even if sometimes it's not in the
same exact field. If I'm on the Health Committee and somebody
else is on a housing committee, I think it's important that people
meet and exchange ideas because you're working for the same
goals, for improvement of our lives.

Now I've become involved in a school advisory committee.
The people who serve on the committee were elected by their
school community. The notice came home from school one day
asking for nominations to be voted on. I was interested in education, as you know, so I put my own name down. Well, no other
parent put a name down and I was elected as representative for that
school! I began to get an idea of how things were going in that
school district. The parent participation was really very low.

Thank goodness I have the kind of husband I have. Very good
natured. I can remember a few times different crises came up and
I'd be at the Health Center, the kids with me, at a meeting and he'd
come home from work with no supper started. He'd pick up the
kids, take them home, start supper. I was still at the meeting.
Never any question. And I have so much material at home I have to

read. I need a library—it's just awful. I've taken the whole dresser. My husband's clothes are jammed in one drawer, instead of the whole dresser he had, and I have papers, pamphlets, minutes in the other drawers.

Going back to the time of the budget cut when you resigned. We really didn't know about budgets before then. Then we got into it and started writing to our representatives as I said. And then, you remember, when some of us went to Washington about funding for the Center? This really opened our eyes more about the government. We realized the big mess about funding. This department and that department. Then we became very interested in the Health, Education, and Welfare bill. Now I find myself always listening to things on the television, that I never listened to before. I used to have no idea what they were talking about.

Now I hear about the President and this bill and that bill. I never had much knowledge before about the President. How he was running things. But now I can look at different things, and say I don't like the way he's doing that—I don't think that's necessary, or this *is* necessary. That's why I say this whole thing has opened up such a world to me.

I've been thinking about doctors a lot and about medical students especially. When I was at that conference in New Hampshire we talked a lot about medical students. We were talking about them coming out to communities. I told them "I don't want you to give me health care because you're not ready for it. I don't want you to give my baby a shot. But I want you to come out and see where I live, walk through the halls that I walk through, walk through the streets. Kick the grass off your feet, and look at the children and people and how we live, and get knowledge. Maybe you won't ever work in a community. But if you do, it's very important and even if you don't, it's important because you should know different parts of life and what's going on."

I told them how very important I felt medical students were. I said, "You're the future. Of course the doctors of today, the older doctors are important too. But I feel you're more important. You're learning, you're the doctor of tomorrow. You're going to save my life. You're going to cure me of cancer. You're going to cure my children. You're going to help me live longer. You're very important."

I'm very strong about medical students coming and really observing what's going on and really talking to people . . . getting an idea. We're not all dirty . . . if we are, find out the reasons why we are. Why we don't take care of ourselves. If that's the case why we don't receive the medical care we should. Why the poor contract this disease or that disease quicker. Probably have more TB cases than other people and don't go to the doctor even though there is a City Hospital.

I imagine there's not too much time that medical schools have to allot to students to go into the community health center, or if there isn't a health center just to visit the community in some way. But take the schools of social service. I think they should spend much more time in the field. Public Welfare I think should spend all their time out there—forget what they learned in the books.

Even if doctors never work in the community they may have some influence later in life. They may become the kind of doctor who sits on boards and makes decisions about people who live in a community like Bracken Field.

I used to want to be a nurse. But I've become more social minded . . . more community minded. When we began talking about and to professionals, the committee people would say. "We are not doctors. We have no intention of running this clinic as a doctor would." But when it comes to social workers we don't say that. We don't have a formal degree. But often we deal with people like social workers do. We deal with people on our level, the poor people in the community. We are those people. And I've come to learn many, many things, probably not as much as social workers; I won't go that far, but I've learned many things. These people have gone years to school, and had years of learning. I have lived what they have learned, I know that if I ever went to work again, I could never take a job typing. I would itch if I was sitting behind a desk and not really being able to get out and see the problems or the progress. I would want a job in the community, talking to people and doing that sort of thing. Being on the Health Committee has really done this.

I really feel that I'm being of service to myself because I learned so much. It's just opened up so many things I didn't know before. People to turn to and different ways of looking at things. But just now I'm not setting my heart on any career, except finishing high school. I'm definitely going to do that some day . . . if I have to take my babies with me.

Martha Maloney —
A West Hill Health Committee Member

Until she was fifty, Martha Maloney devoted herself entirely to the care of her family. A modest woman, she was gratified by the ready acceptance of her ideas at meetings. Her interests and activities grew alongside her increasing involvement in health organization as she began to discover talents and abilities in herself she had not known she possessed.

I'm an only child, and my father died when I was very young. My mother worked and we always were very poor. I didn't have anything really in my background that would bring me into this community health field but possibly psychologically there is one thing that I keep thinking back to . When I was very young, I fell and my mother had to take me to East Huntington Hospital. I had cut my leg. I remember at that time my mother didn't have the money to pay the hospital. She said that she would bring the money the next time she came, and I remember the social worker being actually nasty to my mother. This has alway stayed right with me. Then I had to go back to the hospital all by myself because my mother couldn't take the time off from work the second time. I must have been about nine years old because my father died when I was nine. I remember I wouldn't tell them my name; I was so afraid that because my mother hadn't paid they wouldn't let me in. They asked had I ever been there before and I said no, I hadn't. Now maybe psychologically that's what brought me into the Health Committee.

Then too I have my own children—nine of them. Fortunately they were all healthy children, and I didn't have any great expense with them other than accidents or colds or things like that. For anything that really bothered them I would take them to East City Hospital because I couldn't pay East Children's Hospital's fees.

My husband's a post office worker. We're married twenty-seven years, and in all our twenty-seven years he's never lost a day's work. So it wasn't a case of not having the money, but we had many children. I remember that Mary Ann once was in the East Children's Hospital, and we had to pay part of her bill. We have always had some type of hospitalization insurance. I can re-

member my husband writing to tell them that we would be late with
the payment. They were never very nice to us. They were paid, of
course, in time, but sometimes something would come up so that
possibly one week we wouldn't have enough money to pay them.
All these things might have made me more conscious of health.

Then I've always been mindful that health care is so important, and I've always wanted the best for the children. Maggie had
an appendix once; that was one of the major things that happened
to us, and again I went to East City Hospital. I would have pre-
ferred to go to East Children's Hospital but I knew I could never afford it, and I felt it wasn't fair to my husband. He always worked
hard, and he never drank in his life . . . gave up cigarettes even to
help towards his own good health. It wasn't fair to give him ulcers
which we readily could do over a hospital bill. I myself had a breast
abscess after one of the babies was born and had to go back in the
hospital, and naturally we had run up quite a hospital bill due to the
fact that I had to come home and have penicillin each day at home.
My husband did develop stomach trouble at that time, the poor
fellow. We had to have a doctor come in to see me every other day
and of course all those bills built up and my husband went and got a
loan to pay . . . he always wanted his bills paid . . . to pay off the
doctor and the druggist. You know penicillin was expensive at that
time. I always felt that it was very hard to build up a big hospital bill
and pay it, and then have the father wind up with ulcers and the
mother wind up having a nervous breakdown, and conflict in the
family through nothing but both parents being worried over the
bills. And I have always felt that in this large city we should get the
very best of health care. So I think that would be part of the reason
I became interested in the West Hill Health Committee.

All of my children have always belonged to organizations.
Neither myself or my husband ever have. The children were
always active in Scouts and things like that. For all the years that
they were growing up I actually never left the house. I really am a
very secluded person because all my time was devoted strictly to
them. They were never left with a baby-sitter.

And financially we weren't able to go out. We would enjoy
things together like we'd go to the Museum or . . . my husband's a
a great reader and even if I didn't read, he often would discuss what
he had read with me, and we'd go to the park and enjoy ourselves
that way. We never had a car. I was never discontented that we had
nine children. Of course it was a sacrifice, but neither one of us

ever were selfish. We were always very contented with just what we had, which was, you know, very little.

Racial prejudice? No, I never did have any racial prejudice and I'll tell you why probably. My mother was real Irish, and she worked the hard way. She worked in hotels and she worked in the Theological School. She said that the people she worked with who were the nicest to her were always the black people that she became associated with. My mother was very tolerant, and yet we were brought up in a strict Irish neighborhood. I never did have any prejudice.

As a matter of fact, when Johnny was going to graduate from the eighth grade . . . he had gone to parochial school . . . his father said to me, "We've got to start thinking about sending him to a public school, Martha. He's really in a very closed way, and we have to let him know that there's other people besides Catholics in the world." So I said, "Yes, that a good idea. I'll speak to the Sister." And Sister said, "By all means, get him away from us nuns." Well, he went to Boys High School. I know that many, many Jewish boys go to Boys High. His first day home I said to him, just by way of conversation, I said, "Johnny, are there many Jewish boys in your room?" He turned and looked at me. "I don't know. I wouldn't know one." I felt good about that, I did.

Let me get back to your question on organizations. It's only in the last few years that I started joining organizations. The women's club in our parish was the first thing. Later I joined the Community Action Program and then the West Hill Health Committee that you and Kate and the Health Advisory Group of the Health Center got started. I didn't think I would join but my husband said, "Actually, Martha, I think you should; you probably should get out more now the children are grown because your world will close in on you if you don't." So I agreed, and that was the start of it. My husband works nights. But then again there's always somebody at home . . . Mary Ann or one of the older ones with the children.

I enjoyed the meetings. I found that I was learning a lot myself. . .things that I didn't know about. . .that I was really getting an education in a sort of way by going and exchanging ideas. Very soon after the West Hill Committee really got going, East City Hospital wanted a representative from the committee for their advisory group. I was asked to serve and I agreed. I've been really active in that. I'm not afraid to speak my mind. As I say it has given me an education. Many of the people on the committee never would have met otherwise, and there are a lot of things you learn by meeting different people. It may be just a recipe from somebody else that you never would have gotten if you hadn't been there. And how different people think and how different people have different views than we do. And yet you can see their views. I'm not always in agreement with everything on the Advisory Board, and, just by the same token, everybody isn't in agreement with me either.

I never wanted it to become a social sort of thing. I think that on things like this you can meet with people and exchange your views and get along very well with them. But I don't think it's wise with people that you meet like that, to tell them all the secrets of your family . . . I think that's not good, and I don't think anybody should ever ask secrets of anybody else's family. Even to now, I've known you how many years, and it's only now that I feel that I can ask you how many children you have.

The West Hill Health Committee is progressing well with its plans to start another health center in South West Hill. Other communities are also starting their own health centers.

I feel that the community should have the right to have a say in what they want for their families. I do not think speaking for myself, that I am well qualified to have any control or to have all of it. I think taking care of the people, the patients, should be left entirely to professionals. You could call me a middle-of-the-roader. I feel that people should have something to say in what type of services we're going to have . . . the quality of it . . . I certainly think that if we felt that somebody or some person wasn't what we thought was qualified, we should be allowed to voice our opinion. You will see though, Doctor, that many times you won't find two people who would agree with each other. I don't think that the community is . . . how will I put it . . . all ready. We do have learning to do before we would be able to have control.

I think there should be a partnership. I do think that there is a lot to be learned by the hospitals and professionals also. For so long now the people have been just sort of . . . I won't say nothing, but they have just been sort of numbers. You know, you're given a number and you have to wait. That's certainly very, very disassociated from the community. I do think it's about time that the professionals knew that people are human beings along with being a patient.

Nancy Early —
Chairman of West Hill Health Committee

"I was never important to me" is Nancy Early's assessment of herself before she became Chairman of West Hill Health Committee. A very shy child, fat, the third of nine children, Nancy had no thought of leadership. She moved into the project soon after marriage, and found living there pleasant until most white families had moved out and were replaced by severely disadvantaged blacks. Nancy Early's oldest son was constantly tormented by the project's black children, and she found an apartment outside the project. Two years later the Earlys were forced to return to the project because they could not afford the rent elsewhere.

Membership in the Advisory Health Committee was a catalyst in Mrs. Early's development. I watched with awe her hesitancy change to confidence, her timidity to sureness, her shyness to composure. There will be no turning back.

Having the Health Center here is beautiful. I'm partial to the Health Center—it gives so much help, and it's growing. I think Dr. Will is marvelous, and all the doctors are good. They really understand the community, and the neighborhood aides and the social workers get you help if you really need it. We don't have 24-hour service, but you can get some help, and you don't feel so isolated. I don't know what the project would be like without it. To me it would be hell. I don't think I could stand living there without the Health Center because it's been like . . . what would you call it? A salvation? It's a place that I feel I'm comfortable in and a place I can go to if I need help.

I think I became the Secretary of the Bracken Field Advisory Health Committee shortly after you left. As far as the West Hill Health Committee is concerned, I understood when I became chairman of that committee that it was supposed to be a coordination of the three groups (Bracken Field Health Committee, Model Cities Health Committee and South West Hill Health Committee) into one large group to get better health services for all of the West Hill area. We're hoping that anything to do with health will feed into the large group. We agreed to use the parliamentary procedure that is in Robert's Rules. If the members have agreed to use the

Rules, then they have to use it—that's one of the basic things. One of my biggest things as Chairman is I try to keep putting down their throats that if you have no trust in each other, then you have no committee. And another thing I keep saying in our workshops is that the community people are the strongest voice going. It annoys me when in our Bracken Field meetings they'll open up and talk like nobody's business, and in the West Hill meetings everybody sits like a dumbbell. Unless I say to them, "What's your opinion . . . what's yours . . . ," they won't open up.

Yes, I have got a great deal of satisfaction from being chairman. I wouldn't want to give up the chairmanship. If it came to a vote and election, and I was not re-elected, then I would gracefully step down whether I liked it or not because that's the way to do things. But that doesn't mean I have to like it. I like the role of chairman . . . I like the role of a leader. Not so much dictating to people . . . not so much telling people what to do . . . maybe it's the dependency of people on me that I like . . . I don't know. I just like people, and I like to talk . . . I like to visit . . . I don't care whether the dishes are done . . . I'll go to a meeting.

The people I have met, the doctors and students and community people and everybody . . . I just get a great joy out of meeting people and I really am amazed that people who have a lot of status will ask my opinion, even though I say community people have to feel as though they're important and that they can speak up and their opinion is important. I never thought I was important either, until I found that people were listening to my opinion and asking for it because they sincerely wanted it. When I found this out, then I realized that as a person I was important, and I feel that other community people should feel the same way. They are important and they don't feel it, and I think this is part of what's wrong with our committee. To me the most important thing is to make them feel what I have felt, that it really is exhilarating to feel that Dr. Mann [Associate Director of East Huntington Hospital, through whose good offices the Health Center obtained services for its adult population.] who has so much status, thinks that my opinion as a person is important, and he's not inviting me just because he has to.

The first time I went to the University to talk to dental students, one student really got me upset. He thought it interesting that people on Welfare would question whether they had top quality services. I really got mad and I told him the days of cattle going through a turnstile was gone. Anyway they asked me back this year, and I really can't explain the feeling I had when they asked me back. I didn't think they would, and I was very glad when they did.

I'm seeing one of the social workers at the Health Center once a week now. She said to me that every time somebody gives me a compliment, I knock myself back down again. For instance, she said to me, "That's a beautiful cake," that I made, and I said, "Oh, it's not as good as the one I made such and such a time, you know." She said, "Why, it's a beautiful cake. Next time somebody gives you a compliment, just say thank you. Don't knock yourself back down." I find it very hard to do this. Because I never was important to me . . . I never felt important at home. I was in a shuffle of kids, and everybody had to do what they were told. We had a lot of fun at home, but I never was put into a position where I was the center of attraction. I loved that position, but I was so scared of it. I was very heavy for my size . . . I was called names all my life. When I was going to school, part of my trouble of being a slow learner was that I was afraid to get up and answer. I might be wrong. My father was a very humble person. His feeling was that you don't draw attention to yourself for any reason; but my mother was very outgoing. She always said, "There's a lot of people as good as you, but there's not anybody better." I never thought about what she said till I got into this chairmanship, but then I stopped and thought, "Well, that's right."

I always felt as though I was a good person, you know, and that I was doing right by the kids, but I never felt myself anything but a housewife. Now I feel as though I can give so much more. And I don't mind giving it. Health-wise, not physical health, health-wise as far as the pattern of how health needs are met, the funding and that type of thing, I've learned an awful lot. I always felt before that things were this way because it had to be, and you had to accept it. I find now that you don't have to accept it . . . that you can find other means. You don't have to accept Dr. Cartwright's deal because he says he's Dr. Cartwright. You can stand up and tell him, "That's wrong," if you don't like what he says. "That's wrong, we don't want it, go to the devil, we don't have to take it."

The training we had at the Antipoverty Agency was tremendous. Every one of the committee people should go through some kind of training, I feel. I don't care what it is or what it does to them, whether it develops them as a person or whether it's educational, they need some kind of training. I was in the mold before and I didn't question it. Now I find that people just don't have a thought of their own. They just go along and do what is right. Well, who says it's right? This is what keeps coming up into my mind. I always used to feel that because Dad and Mom said it was right, that it was right . . . because a police officer said it was right . . . a firemen . . . a doctor . . . it was right. But I find now that it's not always so. As a person talking to a doctor about yourself, you might be right and he might be wrong. It's very different now.

When I won Chairmanship of West Hill Committee, I just really sat there and I was afraid to tell Dr. Mann that he's out of order or something like that. You don't have to be nasty, but you can be firm, and I was always afraid. But I'm not afraid any more.

Celia Holder —
Chairman, Advisory Health Committee

Celia, embittered by an unhappy childhood, and burdened in bring-
ing up her own children, some of whom suffered from retardation,
found release and fulfillment in unrelenting work on behalf of con-
sumer participation in health affairs. Her manner, her pointed and
often accusatory statements, her bluntness of approach, upset
many people. But Celia's intelligence and perserverance, and her
complete dedication to the task of consumer development earned
her increasing respect. She became a force on behalf of con-
sumerism far beyond the confines of Bracken Field and her own de-
velopment was as remarkable as the development of the Advisory
Health Committee which she chaired.

I think the committee made me come out of the shell that I was in.
It got me out from my family problems. Maybe that's why I can
cope with an awful lot more as I get older because I have an out.
Everybody needs an out. I think that's one of the reasons why a lot
of the mothers come, because I heard a mother say the other day,
"I'd rather come to these meetings than go home and look at four
walls or listen to a bunch of screaming children." It saves a lot of
their sanity, okay? That's where it helped me. It helped me get
something that I wanted . . . something and some reason to why I
went to work. I went to work to help my family get from under . . .
out of the project. We all dream that some day we'll live
somewhere else, or we'll own our own home . . . which is a lot of
dreams . . . probably never will, but if you stop dreaming, might as
well forget it and die. And every time I face a new wedding an-
niversary, I say, "Oh . . . no further than we were sixteen years
ago."
    Working on the committee developed me to the extent that I
can go out and work on my own and try to help people in other
areas, teach them the things I learned and help guide them in the
right direction so they won't be taken down the drain like a lot of
people have been taken. The Advisory Committee has helped a lot
of mothers mobilize. We have an awful job ahead of us convincing
others that it is our right as American citizens to help take part in
this and that—it isn't up to the individual institution to make decisions on how our life is going to be run. It's a shame that the

Housing Development can't get more people interested enough to push the Housing Authority to really do what they want. There are a few changes but it's a few, very, very dedicated people that have done it.

Years ago when I was just a housewife, that's what I was, and I was happy to be it. Serving on committees didn't mean too much to me. I got interested in the Health Center and the Advisory Committee mostly because of my own children, and what I wanted for them. And then it became that instead of being a nobody, all of a sudden, you've got people saying to you . . . "Oh, you do have something there." How can I explain it? My big mouth. I think that there are a lot of people in projects and in communities that have said in their own mind that this is my life and this is where I stay. But there's a lot of talent there and a lot going on. People in communities aren't stupid. Far from it. Institutions like hospitals and housing authorities have begun to realize that. I think they should definitely take people like myself, and Nancy Early and others and really educate us because if they could do that, and use the resources they have, this would become a very much better country to live in. There are so very few of us, and sometimes we get the feeling that we as individuals are not ready to cope with the institutions. We know the courts aren't doing what they're supposed to be doing, we know housing isn't. That's why I hope the consumer's organization that is now in focus will be a strong body and will be able to stand up and say, "This is it." I'm hoping the institutions don't think that they're going to run it, because as long as I'm sitting on it, the consumers will run it.

I would like to go to school and get more education, which I think I definitely need. I don't have the finances so I don't go. I just struggle to keep going. I really would like to go much farther in my development. It will be in this kind of field but where or what I don't know now. I know that this job of mine won't be my last stop, because I see a lot wrong with it that I'm not happy with. Unfortunately, it starts out as a great thing, but it gets lost in the shuffle. I don't know if I'd like to get involved in politics because I think politicians lie, and I don't like that. Not that I'm the most truthful person in the world, but I believe there has to be a real, real reason for lying. I just can't see politicians going around and saying one thing and doing the opposite. People abuse and use the political field for their own wants and gains.

What I really and truthfully want out of life is a home for my family and more money coming in so that when my children want something like a bike I can give it to them. I don't want to be rich, I just want to live and let live. But at the same time I like this kind of work and I definitely would like to stay in the community organization field.

But it's a very difficult field. It's not a nine to five deal. It's whatever hours you can put in, and it takes a lot away from your family. Unfortunately, I think that a lot of people that are interested in it aren't ready to sacrifice. People ask me, "Why do you sacrifice your children for such a thing?" I don't feel I sacrifice my children because I feel strongly that my children get a lot out of me, because if you don't have a decent community to live in and you're not going to give yourself to the community, then however much you give your children isn't going to help. Maybe if you sacrifice yourself from your children for a while, in the long run your children won't have to live in filth and misery.

Stella Jones

Unlike my treatment of the other narratives, I present the interview with Stella Jones almost in its entirety. I do this because Stella shows so clearly certain traits which are common to all those I interviewed. One of these traits is simple endurance under conditions of chronic stress—the ability to survive day after day without breaking down. Another is a burning sense of injustice and a willingness to fight for the rights of others—the elderly, the bedridden, the sick, the poor, the children. Yet another is compassion, exemplified in the tenderness and care she lavished on the unfortunate people of Sparrow Nursing Home.

Stella is highly intelligent and has a keen sense of humor. She is also impetuous, rash, impulsive. A warm generous person, she is sometimes amused and resigned at her own and others' foibles. On the surface very often brash, opinionated, loud, Stella has a sense of poetry, a love of nature and deep sensitivity. Too many people see only the dark side of Stella—a side she often deliberately presents. My own relationship with her was warm. She, more than most, understood what I was trying to do with the members of the Advisory Health Committee of which she was a member, and she compared my work with them to her own nurturance of the tomato seeds she grew—an apt analogy.

I'm twenty-nine and a half. I was born on a very small island in Maine, and I grew up there. My mother wasn't married. My father was a lobster fisherman who lived on the island. He was married to someone else and had three kids just my own age. I used to spend weekends at their house, but I didn't know he was my father. When I was about ten, he moved away from the island, and I grew up with my grandmother and grandfather on a small farm.

My mother would come in and out, but, like, I couldn't stay with her. We just didn't get along at all, in any way, shape or form. For one thing I have a half-sister who's three years older than I am. Okay. My mother didn't want her. She wanted a boy because she worked on a big farm. My mother does all man's work. I've never seen her with a dress on. They say she's a tough worker. When my sister came along, I guess she decided she'd put up with her; but when I came along that was too much to take because she didn't want two girls—she wanted a boy.

I get this information from one of my mother's sisters, Aunt Fay, a very nice person, a real, real beautiful lady. Most of the people in my family aren't worth a damn . . . they're really bad, evil, narrow-minded, white people, and, you know, no income. They won't change their ideas or opinions on anything, and anybody that's got different opinions is bad. But Aunt Fay is different than that. She's more open than the rest of the family . . . that's not saying too much. I always got along with Aunt Fay, but I could never talk with my mother—I couldn't talk with my grandmother either very much. My grandmother really loves me, but she's a real way-out person. She's eighty-nine, and she raises a great, a huge, great, big garden and a beautiful flower garden, and she has a great big raspberry patch. My grandfather's old . . . he's ninety-three, and he's a caretaker now for these rich people that come up there in the summertime. He takes care of their lawns, sees that their house is okay in the winter time. He still goes to work every day. Doesn't make much money, but it doesn't cost as much there.

Some of the ideas I have about money now is because of the money situation when I was growing up. Because we didn't have any money . . . absolutely no money. But on this island, where you can't get off unless you go on the ferry boat, which is twelve miles across the water to the mainland . . . there isn't anything to spend money on. So you don't need money because everybody owns their own house, and it's not fancy. It's not like city people getting something fancy so the other people have to get something fancy to go along with it. They don't have all that competition and stuff. They grow their own vegetables and they catch their own fish and clams and scallops and lobsters and crabs. In the city they're pushing pollock, and they're pushing mussels, saying, "Oh it's so healthy for you." People up home don't eat that. They throw it away, and they use the pollock for bait. The people in the city don't know enough not to eat it. They eat it because the newspapers say it's good for you.

I was really quite unhappy when I was little. I used to . . . I don't know now if it was just a habit . . . but I used to cry myself to sleep every night. Grammie used to put me to bed when it started to get dark. We had all these trees by my bedroom and she'd say, "Well, the birds are going to bed, so you've got to go to bed, and when the birds get up then you can get up." So I'd go to bed, and I'd just cry and cry . . . I used to do that every night . . . cry, and cry. Now I can't cry, but I used to cry all the time.

I remember telling Grammie I wanted to go to school, but she said I couldn't go till I was old enough. When I started going to school I was so skinny, sixty-eight pounds. Grammie finally took me to the doctor checking to see if I could gain more weight. And then I hated school. I hated to sit down and try to apply myself to studies. Like I've always wanted to be outdoors, doing something outdoors. I'd walk back home for lunch—it was about two miles— and then walk back up to school. There's a big cow pasture which goes almost all the way around the whole school, and I used to sit there in class and watch the cows with these cow bells on them . . . clang . . . clang . . . watch the cows. I really love cows. I'd do anything but study. If I'd been down in the city, I'd never in hell have finished high school, but there's nothing else on the whole damn island to do but go to school; so you really don't have a choice.

The school was boring as hell. The teachers were all terrible. The books were old, old, rackety books. The teachers were old people. Like the town, of course, don't pay very much money for teachers. People down here in the city think a small class and ev- erybody knowing everybody is the best possible learning situation, but if you've got an old dead teacher that couldn't give a damn less, you're not helped to get curious. I think everybody naturally has it in the beginning, but you have to know how to expand it. Every- where you go it's discouraged.

I love basketball. I was the captain of the basketball team in the sixth, seventh, eighth, freshman, sophomore, junior, senior year. But like I can't spell. I can't remember numbers, and I make it a point not to remember numbers because they just confuse my mind, and I can always look them up so why remember them? My half sister that's three years older than I am she can spell any word anything. So I grew up with this real complex about my sister who was so damn smart and I was so damn dumb, and I've still got a complex.

My mother graduated from high school. She was historian, third in her class. My sister graduated from high school. She was historian, third in her class, and I graduated high school, third in my class, historian. But then, you see, there were only eight people in my class; so when you figure it out, you had to be pretty damn dumb to get left out.

I didn't always get along with Grammie because she was strict in her ways, though she wasn't strict with me. As a matter of fact my grandmother believed in freedom, but she was narrow-minded. And all the time my mother was in the background, and every time

she would come in the house it was always a battle, an instant battle. Like two fighting cocks that have just got to fight each other
every time they see each other. I always thought she was picking
on me, she'd always find something wrong. For a long time I used
to have all these bad feelings about her inside of myself, and I'd just
walk away and ignore her. Finally, I said, "Look, the hell with this,
I'm not taking this kind of crap from anybody." And then I re-
belled.

I decided that I had been around enough at home, so when I
was eleven I started working for some summer people as a maid in
their house, and I worked there every summer after that and went
to school. There were three hundred natives on the Island in 1958.
With the summer people it would go to one thousand and five hundred. The A's camp up there every summer, the B's, that
Republican Senator that retired a few years ago, he comes up every
summer. Dr. C., a famous communist, comes up there and Dr. D.,
a famous New York brain surgeon, goes there . . . all these rich
people. And all the natives take care of their houses.

I stopped living with my grandmother when I was fifteen. The
summer people that I worked for had a little cabin for the maid
quarters, and there was a breezeway connected to the house. That
summer I was working there as a cook, and they told me I could
live there for the rest of the winter if I wanted to. So I stayed there
two years. It was good. I was alone. I didn't have to worry about
nothing. I had three cats and a dog with me because I really like
animals, but that's all.

In 1958 when I graduated, I worked home that summer, and
then in September I came down with people, whose kids I knew, to
live with them in Greentown as a mother's helper. I needed a job,
and I wanted to get off the island.

Coming down by train to East City, I was overwhelmed. To
top it off I had a very thick accent. People on the island talk in a
kind of different way than even people on the mainland talk. People
on the mainland can't understand people on the island. In Greentown or in East City, I'd go into a store to ask for something and
the people would say, "What?" I was very, very shy.

Like I had never even seen a policeman before. On the island
we had a deputy sheriff, who was my uncle, but he didn't wear a
uniform. He never did anything. A few people bootlegged, but he
did it too. The Fish and Game Wardens came around sometimes. I
was petrified of police. All the time I was growing up, my

grandmother took the East City Post which went defunct in 1956. She would never get the local Maine papers. In the evenings, my grandmother sat on a chair in the kitchen, and my grandfather lay on the couch discussing the newspaper. That was when I read about police.

They would like to discuss politics. I remember it used to bug the hell out of me, but if the headlines would have something about Russia it would be, "Them goddam Russians . . . what do them Russians think they're doing . . ." Something about Charles de Gaulle . . . "That goddamn Frenchman . . . what's he think he's doing." No matter what it was about, she'd be swearing and cussing. If it was an American Indian, she'd be cussing about the Indians. Later on it got to be the black people, and she'd be cussing about them.

On the same hand, my grandmother's teaching me that I should love everybody. "Stella, you must love everyone." She repeats this over and over to me, that I should love everyone completely, love people. But on the other hand if you didn't come from that island in Maine, then you were no damn good.

Like my Aunt Fay ended up marrying a guy from Rocksea where the ferry boat goes to . . . a town of about twenty thousand. Because he came from Rocksea, my grandmother'd say, "Ya, ya, ya, that Fay married that city slicker down there." He moved to the island and became the postmaster. He's the only man in town that wears a white shirt . . . and he's a city slicker!

They had two kids . . . Aunt Fay wasn't supposed to have any children because she had a very bad accident when she was a teenager, but she wanted children, and she had two about five years apart. I used to take care of them.

When the little girl was thirteen, in 1964, she woke up one night with a sore throat. She gargled with listerine, and they put her back to bed. Seven o'clock in the morning she woke up and couldn't talk. She was freezing and her fingernails were blue. There's no doctor on the island—you have to go to Rocksea. In the summertime the rich people bring over their own doctor. The natives don't use the summer people's doctor much . . . I mean there's no law about it but an unspoken rule. Aunt Fay was very worried about the girl, and she called the summer doctor. It was on a Sunday morning. The doctor was very nasty and said there was nothing wrong—laryngitis was all.

"Well she's having trouble breathing," said Aunt Fay.

"No, it's your imagination." The doctor got up to go.

"Are you going to leave?"

"I'm going to church—I'll be back after church."

About eight o'clock she died. She just died. Uncle Sam started doing mouth to mouth resuscitation and doing all kinds of things he didn't even know how to do, but he couldn't bring her back to life.

They sent the body over to Rocksea for an autopsy. It was pneumonia. Aunt Fay never really got over it. Uncle Sam aged tremendously. The little boy that was left, he's turned into a hippie.

Anyhow to get back to me. I went to work for this family in Greentown. I couldn't get along with them at all. Oh, I couldn't get along with that lady. Mind you, I wanted to work, and I worked very hard, but the more I worked, the more they piled it on me. The husband was nice, and the kids were nice, but she came from a wealthy family in the Mid-West, and she put on all these airs.

Finally I left there and went to work in the next town for a while. The lady was pregnant. Matter of fact she had the baby the night I got there. She wanted someone to stay in the house for a couple of weeks while she was in the hospital. She was German. Her husband was from England and talked that real kind of way that some English people talk. I couldn't understand him. I couldn't understand anything his wife said. Neither one of them could understand me. Their little five year old girl, Moppet, could understand everything. She got German. She got English. She could talk to everybody. We all used to talk through Moppet . . . she was a real sharp kid.

He raised Black Angus bulls for a hobby. They had a flock of guinea hens, and a flock of ducks and a flock of geese, and a couple of pigs and all this stuff. It was the first time I ever lived on a farm that had money enough to have all the stuff you need. And it was beautiful. I was hired for two weeks and was talked into taking it, but I stayed there six months. I loved it. They didn't hardly pay me anything because that wasn't the agreement, but I wasn't working there for money anyhow. I loved it there, and I loved the little girl, and then the baby came home, and the mother wasn't well; so I used to take care of the baby, and I got really fond of the baby. This was the first time that I ever took care of a little baby. And it grows on you.

At that time, my older sister, Helen, came down here to East City with her boyfriend who was from the next island to ours. He was a lobsterman there. He got a job in East City as a janitor, superintendent of a building. That way you get your apartment free. They were supposed to get married. I don't think they ever really did get married, but they lived together, and they've got a couple of kids now. They get along good. She is huge, wears a size fifty-two bra, and he's just the same size . . . two great, big fat people. What a pair! She bosses him all around. I used to come in and see them once in a while, and when I left my job with the family, I rented an apartment with them and moved into East City. But first I went home for the summer, and got a job at the Rocksea Hospital as an assistant dietitician.

I liked the hospital and my job. The hospital kitchen was very strict about the people on special diets, what they didn't eat was measured and recorded. I got interested in hospitals when I was there, and in sick people, and the complete lack of doctors and that kind of thing on the island. If you had a serious accident, the coast guard would send over a hospital boat, but on the whole people got little care, and very few people seemed to get sick. But like there's woodcutters up there, and fishing is dangerous. And most fishermen drink. I mean they're half stewed most of the time, but that's just the way they do their work.

You really have to be drunk to go out on that damn water. Like, I grew up there. I love the water, the ocean. I like to sit on the bank somewhere and just stare at the water and meditate. And all that movement of the water washing up on the shore, every single time that water is different. I wish to hell I was back there looking at that water. But I get sea-sick. I can't swim—I'm petrified. Most of the people who grew up on the island can't swim. Most are petrified of the water. You grow up to respect that water. It's cold, freezing. The only people who swim up there are the summer people . . . they don't know any better. Mainers don't have too much respect for the rich people. They come up there, and they drive like hell around the island, they're out to let off steam for the summer, but for people who live there all the time it looks kind of asinine.

So working in that hospital situation really started me to thinking about all the health ideas and everything. See, my teeth were very bad . . . like all the time I was growing up, I never went to a dentist. And like most people up home have very bad teeth. They have terrible teeth. So right after I graduated and went to Greentown, as soon as I was earning money every week, the first thing I did was go to this dentist to get my teeth fixed. I went all the time I was living in Greentown and as a matter of fact, I would have left the job sooner, but I was going to the dentist till I got my teeth completely fixed. And that took the money I earned.

Well after the summer I spent at the Rocksea Hospital, as I said, I rented the apartment in East City from my sister and her husband, and I answered an ad in the paper for training as an aide at East General Hospital. "We'll train you . . . pay you while you're training." One part of the hospital was for the rich folk—Smart House. I worked there, and they thought I was a maid, I guess. All the rich people . . . and hardly any of them were sick. They all came in to get over a hang-over, or lose five pounds, or some damn stupid thing, and sit up in a big fancy hospital bed, and use the stationery, and make you run up and down and answer the light, but they don't really want anything.

The aides do most of the running up and down answering the lights because the aides do the really important work of being nice to the patients. The nurses come in all efficient and everything when that's necessary, and they have all the know-how, but like some of them can't get along with the patients. And even those patients that aren't sick and just putting on, you still have to know how to get along with them. Anybody that's going to act like they do got to be wrong in the head, so you have to take that into consideration; where they're mentally sick you just go along with it, you know. So I worked there . . . oh golly, I worked there a long time.

I couldn't understand some of the things that were going on. It was such a fancy hospital with such a good name, but those people who were all supposed to be on special diets, the kitchen didn't take any care of them. Somebody's supposed to be on a low sodium diet or something . . . half the time the plates would get mixed up. "Oh what the hell. What the hell." And in Smart House, anything the patients wanted they'd write out on the menu. Anything a patient wanted they could have, no matter what diet they were on. The doctor would say, "Well if they want it, give it to them." They didn't care. They just put them on a special diet just for the hell of it, just to say they did something, but they didn't pay any attention to it. I couldn't understand it because the Rocksea Hospital was so particular about it.

Then I went onto night shift in the intensive care unit. It was a very good experience, and those patients were really sick. When you're on eleven to seven, you get to do much more, and you don't have so many people jumping down your back and much more responsibility. The nurse and doctors were very good, and I really liked that. It's amazing to see some of the patients come in there like on the way out, and in two weeks they'd go home. I stayed there until I left to go to the Guild School for licensed practical nurse training.

I was going to nurses school . . . I had to work, too, and live in the school. And I couldn't get along with those people at the school. I couldn't get along with them because of the very idea that what they were teaching was completely irrelevant to what a nurse needs to know. I had an idea of what needed to be taught, but they didn't have any idea of teaching it. This nutritionist in the LPN school, oh I'd get so *mad* at her . . . called her all kinds of names . . . I got kicked out of school.

This nutritionist was teaching us . . . "The most important thing you really have to know about nutrition is how to make good coffee. If you know how to make good coffee, you're going to put your patients at ease, and then everything else will follow naturally. And the way you make good coffee is this way."

I swore. I couldn't stand it. I was tired, working and going to school. I was *fed up* with that damn school. "The most important thing that a nurse needs to know if she's going to be any damn good is how to stop wasting time, get things done that need to be done and get it done quick." That's what I said. So they kicked me out of school. I'd been there five months. I really should have stuck it out . . . see, if I was an LPN now . . .

I had absolutely no money. I didn't have any place to live because I had sublet my apartment. I didn't have a job. I took my stuff over to my sister's apartment, and then I just walked out of there . . . I didn't get along with her too good. And I wasn't going to impose on her. When I get in really bad shape, I go down to the point and sit and look at the water. I started walking along the jetty, and way out in the middle, too far for me to see him clearly, I saw a guy. There was something about this guy . . . he looked real cute. The closer I got, the cuter he looked. He was black.

I guess I should tell you first about another guy I met before this one. It was when I was working at East General Hospital. I had bumped into a guy in East City. He used to come by my house in the evenings and play records and stuff, and he'd drive me to work. He was a nice guy but crazy . . . nutty. I wasn't really going with him, we were friends. He took me down one Fourth of July to hear a jazz band that he thought real groovy. It was in a rather bad place, and it was jam packed with dancing, and the guy who was playing the sax was black and so *cute* I was just attracted to him. So anyway, I spent the night with the jazz musician. He's a good musician . . . I really fell for that guy. Three days later I got a call from some health department telling me I had gonorrhea.

Of course I went for treatment. I was petrified. I really flipped out. So anyway, that's the couple of experiences that I had. But those guys didn't really mean anything.

So, anyway, I was going down the jetty and this guy was fishing. The only damn thing I know is fish. I asked him what kind of fish he had, and he said he didn't know. This guy sitting out there fishing . . . he doesn't know nothing about fish. The guy was really attractive to me; so, okay, we spent a whole week together. I sat there and talked to him, we went back and had some fried clams and stuff, and then we went to his place, and I stayed with him. And he was a good guy.

It's funny how you pick up some really weird people if you're in the frame of mind to do that. There was sexual attraction. He was young, I was young then. He was very dark, very quiet, from the South. But there was one thing I couldn't understand about him. See people up home very seldom take a bath. Like in my grandmother's house, all the time I was growing up, they only had running cold water. Most people there don't have bathtubs, and they just wash with a washcloth, and they're just not clean. But they don't have lice. And they don't have cockroaches. They keep their houses quite clean and neat, and they do their laundry and hang it outdoors. So when I came to the city I took a bath in the morning . . . I took a bath at night. It was a big treat to me.

This guy had a room on North Avenue. His little room was filthy. The apartment house was full of roaches . . . a mouse and everything. But like he would come out of there looking spick and span. His pants were pressed like he just came out of the dry cleaners. And he didn't *do* anything. He didn't work . . . he didn't do anything. I had never met anybody who didn't work. Up home everybody works all the time. I couldn't figure the guy out. I haven't yet, and I've met a lot of people like him since. I can't understand it. But it's a fact of life around the city. A lot of things in the city I haven't been able to understand.

Okay after I left this fellow, the girl who was in my apartment left, and I moved back in. I got a job working in the Sparrow Hospital nights and a part-time job working at Burns Mail Order in the day. The Sparrow was a chronic disease hospital, but it was like a nursing home. It was pretty dirty, badly run, incompetent staff, not enough anything. Too many patients.

They gave me the second, third, fourth and fifth floor patients . . . there were sixteen patients on a floor. Sometimes one nurse on the floor, sometimes a nurse and a helper. Kitchen's in the basement. Most of the patients are considered senile . . . questionable. Most are covered with bed sores. Most are tied to the bed on their ankles and their wrists. Most have got lice. Most don't have anybody that comes in to see them. It's a really bad hospital . . . nursing home . . . pig pen . . . it would be a bad pig pen.

I like old folks. I like my grandmother and grandfather, and I associate old folks with them. When I went on nights, I had the top floor. There was a guy on the top floor, an alcoholic, an old duffer. They tell me, "That's Alfred . . . he's violent . . . you have to really be careful with Alfred," they said. "When Alfred starts raving and raving, you just have to be very firm with him. If you need any help, call the cops." The thing with Alfred was that he'd wake up in the middle of the night. I looked in his record, and the man always worked nights. So he had a hard time sleeping nights. He'd wake up, and he'd yell "Coffee," on the top of his lungs and all the other nurses would go in and try to shut him up. I said I wasn't going to do that. If the man wants coffee, I'll have coffee ready and give him all the coffee he wants. He used to like a lot of sugar in it. I'd bring the coffee and the sugar and get it ready so when he woke up and wanted his coffee, I'd take it right into him. Look the man wants coffee, give him coffee. That's a simple solution, much simpler than shutting him up. I'm sure he didn't get enough to eat in the daytime.

When I went on the floor, as soon as the nurse left, the first thing I'd do was untie everybody, and loosen their sheets and put their feet on pillows. In the morning I had a mad scramble going around and tieing them up again because I'd have got hell if they knew I was doing that. Those patients needed exercise. They didn't need to be tied down in bed. They needed to get up. So when

Alfred wanted to get up in the middle of the night, I'd let him get up. I used to go in there, turn on all the lights and get the patients up. I know they used to think I was a pain, but I knew they had to stay in bed in the daytime because I worked the day shift before I worked the night shift. It used to make me mad.

It used to get me really upset seeing all them poor patients. It really bothered me . . . all these damn people in this whole damn world, all this stuff going on . . . it makes you wonder. So like Alfred, he'd get up in the night and go to the bathroom. But he'd never *use* the bathroom. They all said, "He's senile, he's senile." He wasn't senile. He just wanted somebody to talk to him. He'd go to the exit down the stairway to the laundry hamper, and he'd always use the laundry hamper to urinate in. All the people used to get mad at him for doing that. I'd just go talk to him, while he's standing there peeing. Sometimes I used to get him to help me with the other patients. And what the hell, if he wants to pee into the dirty clothes, anyway they're going to get washed, let him pee in it. I'm not going to argue with him.

When I was working at the Sparrow Hospital nights, I had this part-time job working over at Burns during the day. I met a guy working there named Noel Johnson. He was black, he was tall, very quiet, very homely . . . one eye crooked. I was working on the eighth floor filling orders and I hated it . . . I hated it. And all the people working there were hateful people. It was very, very busy. And it was hot . . . oh I had a terrible time there. At that time they had hired a lot of Cuban refugees, and they were doing all the work. Little short people, skinny, tough as hell, they carried those great big boxes. The others were resentful of them because they were doing more but the Cubans felt they had to do more to keep their jobs.

This Noel Johnson used to help me. They had seven digit numbers, and you were supposed to keep all these numbers in your mind and get to know where everything was; so when you had to get something, you could run right over where it was and pick it up. I can't remember numbers, period. I do not remember phone numbers or any other numbers. So he was helping me. He had developed a good friendship with some of the Cuban people, and I developed a good friendship with him, and he turned into Danny's father. He was married, a Catholic, had two kids, and his wife had recently separated from him and moved back to New Jersey. Before that she was a nurse's aide, and I knew her a bit. Then she moved back to her home, and I started going out with her husband.

And then I got pregnant with Danny . . . I really wanted to . . . I wanted Danny, you know. I wanted to have a boy, and I kept saying, "Well, if it's a girl . . ."

Noel talked to me. But I said, "Noel, I want to have a little boy . . . I want him to be just like you, and I want to bring him up." Noel's a very reasonable type of person where I'm not particularly. He told me, "Well you think you do, but you really don't. You don't know all the problems involved, and you're going to end up going on welfare." I didn't know what welfare was . . . I knew vaguely, you know, but not really . . . oh my. And I said, "Well I do . . . I want to have a baby." We argued about this for about two years. I really cared for Noel. He was by last night . . . he comes by a couple of times a week . . . comes by on weekends to see Danny and Derrick. He takes them places, and sometimes he takes them to his home. He's back with his wife, and sometimes he brings his other kids in to see them.

This black-white thing. I was talking to a black friend, who's getting a degree in psychology, about it the other day. White girls going with black guys and white guys with black girls . . . that kind of thing. He asked me "Would you just go with black men?" I said, "No. I don't just go with black men. I go with a certain kind of people that I have an attraction to . . . a certain kind of people that I can talk with. They have to have a certain quality which I really cannot label, and the only people that I ever find that have this is black men. I don't find it in white men. Most white men I know are too self-centered . . . too concerned about earning a buck to look at the human side of it." And maybe it's because most of the black people you meet, men you meet in the city who have come up the hard way, understand little kids that have gone through the same thing. That might be part of it.

When I was about six months carrying Danny, I was very big. I mean fat. Like the doctor was telling me, "You can't gain any more weight, it's not good for the baby." (My legs would swell up and my feet.) I'd tell him, "Look, I'm going to gain as much weight as I can because I'm going to have me a healthy baby, and then they'll see that old skinny kid . . . " All the time I was growing up, I was real skinny, and I said, "I'm not having me no kids like that. My kid's going to be big and fat."

I would never go for my check-ups, you know, for months I wouldn't go. Noel is a real bug on health, and he would insist that I go for my check-ups. I'd make him go with me . . . down to East

City Hospital; you go through that and that's bad. I was getting involved in the race problem. I got to know what social workers are, and they make you feel terrible. They make you feel like you're no damn good and all that kind of stuff. All the whole time I was working.

After four months at the Sparrow Hospital, I went to work at the Tate Hospital as a nurse's aide. They put me on the infectious disease floor. It was terrible . . . I hated working there. Cap and gown . . . all that rigmarole. But one good thing I ran into there were the nurses they were bringing over from Ireland. They were efficient, they put the American nurses to shame. They were not fooling around, they knew what the hell they were doing and they worked. And they answered lights and didn't think they were better than anybody else. And like all the time I was growing up, I had Irish people rammed down my throat since I was born. Everybody in my family, everybody on the island is Irish. I finally decided to hell with everybody that's Irish . . . I can't stand Irish people. I had heard they were so damn good for so long I just finally decided, well, the worst people in the world, no matter how bad anybody else is, has got to be Irish. So when I started working with the Irish nurses, I decided there's got to be two kinds of Irish people. Those ones that have just come from the old country, they're good, but these ones that have been here too long, forget them.

When I started getting too big with Danny, I had to leave Tate, and I went to work at the Shortwood Nursing Home in Brooktown. It looked like a beautiful fancy house . . . you come in the front door and the floors are all waxed, and it looks so clean, beautiful . . . yeah, yeah, yeah. Yeah, you go in there at eleven o'clock at night and really look at the place, and what you see is really bad. Not as bad as Sparrow Hospital, but bad. They didn't take good care of the patients. I worked there till Danny was born.

The doctors told me he was supposed to be born in June. Then they said August. They didn't know when he was going to be born, and I just kept getting fatter and fatter. Like I went from one hundred and eighteen pounds to one hundred and sixty-eight pounds. I worked up till about a week before he was born at the end of July. So then I had Danny.

I had arranged with a girl who lived across the street from me and who had a three year old girl herself, to look after Danny when I went back to work. Okay. Fine. I went back to work at Tate Hospital a month after Danny was born.

Noel paid the rent for the month I wasn't working, but like I wasn't getting along with him, and in September I said, "Out . . . go, shoo man . . . make it." He'd come by to see Danny, but as far as he and I was concerned, no, no more. Now we have a relationship where I tolerate him and he tolerates me; he acts like he's Danny's and Derrick's father (of course he isn't Derrick's father). We're just like two people who are divorced, or separated and keep this far apart.

The day I went back to work it was hot as hell. Six o'clock in the morning I had to get Danny up, give him his bath and take him over to the girl's house because I had to be at work at seven. I was worried sick about him. At two o'clock there was a terrible thunderstorm. I thought, "I bet she's out in the thunderstorm with Danny, I bet she's out." I just knew it. I got home as quick as I could. It was still raining, and she's standing on the sidewalk with Danny, and she got on him a pink woolen sweater, and pink mitten things, and pink booties and these heavy clothes, and I just blew my stack—"What the hell you got those clothes on him for?" I got a real thing about over dressing babies. I think they need to have air (as bad as the air is around here) circulating around their body. "Why did you put all those damn clothes on him?" "Oh my goodness," she says, "You didn't bring enough clothes over, so I put some of the clothes on him my baby had before." Oh I blew my stack . . . I blew my stack.

I didn't go back to work. I called them up and said, "I'm sorry . . . " For two months I looked for a decent baby-sitter. I'm paying my rent, and I didn't have hardly any money for food. I couldn't get help from my family. When I was about six months pregnant, my mother came to visit my sister, and she and I got into a huge fight because she carried on like crazy and told me I had to give up this black bastard for adoption.

"No, I don't intend to."

"You *have* to."

"I'm not doing it."

I didn't raise my voice or anything, I just turned around and walked out. She hit me a couple of times.

This period in my life when Danny was born, I really began to realize what being hungry is. When you got somebody else you're taking care of, that's when you begin to realize . . . you can always find something somewhere if you're by yourself, but when you have a little baby, there's baby food and everything else. I was very

particular what I was feeding him. Danny didn't like baby food. He
just spit out baby food. Noel would be up to the house, ''Well, you
don't know how to feed babies.''

Like Noel taught me how to diaper. I had diaper service for
Danny until he was six months old. ''No germs around my baby,'' I
said. ''No baby of mine's going to have diaper rash.''

To look back on it is funny, but I was a nervous wreck at the
time. Every time he'd cry, I'd be out of my mind. Of course he was
healthy. If Danny had been the sick one instead of Derrick, I probably would never have got through . . . I was so nervous. It's
funny, but he was the first thing of my own that I ever had. Later
when I put him in nursery school, it was really hard, really difficult
to do. I think most people, particularly unmarried people, with
their first child have a very difficult time.

Mothers ought to be given enough money to live on, but they
don't have to go to work to get money enough to buy a twenty-four
inch console color TV that goes from one end of the room to the
other. That's not benefitting that baby one damn single bit. You
don't have to have an eight hundred dollar picture on your walls.
You don't have to have an eight-speaker stereo set with speakers in
every room. That baby give a damn less. I might choose some
fancy stuff myself, but not at the expense of saying, ''Okay, I have
to work to have all this stuff because it's nice.'' Not at the expense
of the baby. To hell, it ain't worth it. I had to work to pay the rent
and get food for Danny.

So I put an ad in the paper, and the first person to answer was
a little old lady from Maine with one arm deformed, but I hired her.
She was the only one of the people that answered the ad that came
up to my expectations. Then I went back to Tate Hospital. She
stayed on till Danny got so heavy that she really didn't feel safe,
and she thought she might drop him. And then I got pregnant with
Derrick which was complete, absolute accident. It was terrible . . .
a really bad situation.

I'd gone on the night shift. I'd put Danny to sleep in the carriage, and then take him to the janitor's daughter who also lived in
the building. She was married and had a two year old daughter. In
the morning after work, I'd pick him up. At that time Danny would
be awake most of the day, and by this time I had spoiled Danny
bad. I had this thing like, I'd take him out for walks in the carriage

every day . . . no matter how tired I was, I'd take him because I figured he should be out in the air. I walked and walked with him for miles. I got really tired working all night, and I lost a lot of weight. I was really exhausted, pooped, and then I got pregnant on top of that. It happened this way.

One day I took my laundry to the laundromat which was right in the next building, and I met this nice looking guy standing by the mailboxes in my building. I talked to him for a minute, and he said he was waiting for this other tenant. When I came back from the laundromat, he was still waiting. I said to him, "Look, I know the lady that runs this building, and she don't like black people in this building." I meant very well. Teach me to mind my own business. I said to him, "She sees you hanging around out there, she's going to call the cops, and you're going to be down at that jailhouse before you know what the hell you're doing. If you're waiting for that girl, you'd better wait in my apartment until she gets home." He said no, but I said I thought he'd better or he'd get into trouble. So he came to my apartment . . . we got talking . . . he was from Jamaica . . . and he spent the night. He was a pre-med student at the University. I saw him like two or three times after that, and then I up and got pregnant. How could I get pregnant? You know, I really didn't want to . . . and I couldn't accept it. I didn't go to the doctor and have it verified till I was five months along. I was closing my eyes to it all along. Then I really got sick. I was exhausted. And finally ended up going on welfare.

Well I went on welfare, and then I moved again. Somebody sub-let an apartment to me for three months. When they were due back, I couldn't find another apartment. I had to be out—they were coming back—but I couldn't find one. So people, hippies that lived on Orchestra Road, in the basement, let me live with them for a while. Then this hippie girl and I took an apartment down beside the railroad tracks. She left a little while after we moved in and went to California. Hitch-hiked out. I wish I could really be like that, but I can't. I mean, she just picked up her baby, who was the same age as Danny, and said, "Well I think I'll go back to California." She couldn't find one of the baby's shoes—the baby had one shoe on—and she picked up and went to California. I mean, with no money and just a thumb ride . . . how people do that I don't know . . . I could never do that. Because I have to kind of know where I'm going to sleep tonight. But she did it. People do it.

They have guts, or they don't have brains, they've got something or they're missing something, I can't figure it out.

So then I had this apartment to myself and I was pregnant with Derrick. When I was pretty far along with Derrick, I went to the Welfare Home for Children and they said they'd take Danny until I came home from the hospital with Derrick. The doctor said I was about to deliver . . . Okay. So they put Danny in a foster home for twelve days. Twelve days I went out of my mind worrying about Danny. It was at Christmas time, and like I was going crazy. I finally went out there, and I said, "Look, I'm very sorry, I haven't had the baby yet. You have to give me Danny."

"No, no we won't do that."

"What the hell you mean you won't do it. You just give me Danny."

"Well you come out tomorrow and get him."

I tell you doctor, I went through hell. I finally got Danny. They brought him back from the foster home and I got him home. First thing I checked his fingernails. They hadn't clipped his fingernails. They were dirty. His bottom . . . he'd had a B.M. . . . they hadn't washed his bottom right. He wasn't clean. They put clean clothes on him, but they hadn't kept him clean. Well, that was my dealings with that particular institution.

Now I'm on their board. But I have some questions about it. I've questions about who verifies foster care. Who says that this home or that home is fit to put other people's kids in for a period of time? Who makes the judgment, and on what reasons do they make that judgment? There's more important things than thoroughly washing his buttocks with Phisohex, which I used to do. I mean there's more important things than that in bringing up kids. But that's a little bit part of it. If you're neglecting that, then maybe you're going to be neglecting the other things, too. Or maybe you've got so damn many people in the house you can't take completely care of all of them, but something's got to be figured out there. And then, again, you've got a whole lot of kids, and you haven't got enough foster homes. So I took Danny home with me and, of course, that night I had Derrick.

I was home alone, and the pains started like about midnight. I said, "Well, shit, I can't go to the hospital." When I was carrying Danny, my sister told me she'd had her girls down to East City Hospital, and she told me, "Look, don't go to the hospital till the last minute because it's bad down there on the maternity ward." I had been to the hospital for check-ups because I had RH negative blood. I would go down every two weeks . . ., because I was worried about the baby, and because I wasn't feeling so hot myself. In this pregnancy I wasn't sure of anything. With Danny I had a very positive attitude. So when I was about to deliver Derrick I said, "Well, I can't have him at night time and I'm not going to the damn hospital anyway." Okay, so it was hurting . . . it was hurting.

Soon after I had moved to East City, I had got the use of a little garden allotment where I used to grow vegetables. While I was pregnant with Derrick, I met a black fellow, Melville, who also had a garden out there. He was much older than I was and a bachelor. He liked kids. He used to come down and see me sometimes, help me out and bring me home from my garden. I didn't have a telephone and not much furniture. Four o'clock in the morning I put on my coat . . . it was December 31st. I walked about a mile to use a pay phone, and I called up Melville. "Look, Melville, I'd like to have you come over to the house because I don't feel good, and I don't want to be alone."

"Well, do you want me to take you to the hospital?"

"No, I don't want to go to the hospital till morning, but I don't really want to be alone either."

"Okay."

I walk back to the house, and a damn guy comes along and tried to pick me up. You know, I just carried on like . . . I'm in my nightgown . . . I had my coat over . . . and this guy in this great big fancy car . . . They just cruise around and pick up people down there. This is a big prostitute place down there, and that guy made me so damn mad . . . something's got to be done about those guys.

So anyway I got home, and Melville came over. "Well I'm going to take you to the hospital." He'd never seen anybody that was about to deliver, and like he's an older guy, and he was scared. I wasn't scared, but it was hurting, and my water had broken, and Danny was still in there asleep.

I said, "Well, I don't want to talk about going to the hospital."

"Look, I'm either going to take you to the hospital," he said, "Or I'm going home and go to bed because I'm not going to sit here and listen to you cry."

"Well, go home . . . I thought you were going to be some help, but if you want to go home, damn it, go home."

So he went home. Six o'clock in the morning, the baby was coming, and I was crying. There's this old maid living next door to me, a school teacher, she heard me crying and came in. She went and called the police, and Derrick was born in the paddy wagon, going to the hospital. She stayed with Danny until the police took me into the hospital. They came back, got Danny and admitted him in the hospital.

Because Derrick was born before I got to the hospital, it was a dirty birth, and they didn't put him in with the other babies, and I couldn't go in and see him. Then the doctor came in. Of course I didn't have any anesthesia. The doctor was very nice, and he wanted me to sign a paper for a blood transfusion for Derrick.

When I lived on Xavier Street, I was going to the Jehovah's Witnesses and before that, before I had Danny, I was going to a Christian Science Church. I'm not very religious, but a part of their things I could really associate with. And part of the Jehovah Witnesses' whole business against blood transfusions goes along somewhat with the Christian Science thing. Besides I was against blood transfusions. When I worked at Tate, I'd seen some of those patients come in there and go down to the blood bank, and they say, "Oh hell, we haven't got any of that kind of blood . . . some of this is outdated . . . we'll give it to him anyway . . . he's probably going to die." I don't think they'd get away with it on the day shift, but on the night shift they do that. So I had a bad feeling against blood transfusions, and when the doctor asked me to sign the paper, I refused. "I'm not signing this form. You're not giving no baby of mine no blood transfusions."

"Well, we feel we have to. He's turned jaundiced."

"Well, all the time I was coming in here, you kept testing my blood, and you said there wasn't going to be nothing wrong with this baby. I was in here two days ago, and you promised me there wasn't going to be nothing wrong with this baby. I'm not having no blood transfusions whether you want to do it or not." I was under the impression that if a patient only needs one transfusion, then he doesn't need any. You either need a whole lot, or you don't need none . . . one is worse than none. I guess this is where a little bit of knowledge can really get you screwed up because I didn't know what I was talking about, but I thought I did. Then the doctor told me, "An hour after you came in we transfused him," I was upset. But they'd gone ahead and did it.

Derrick was a tall and skinny baby. Of course, all the time I was comparing him with Danny who was always fat. His skin has a different tone to it then Danny's, and sometimes he looks jaundiced, and I imagine the boy is sick. With him it's been one sickness problem after another. You know, Danny has always been a behavior problem. Derrick's not a behavior problem at all. And he's very smart. Smart as hell. Danny'd much rather raise hell than he would to apply himself to anything, but Derrick's smart . . . he's keen. There isn't any smart people in my family, and so everybody's kind of proud of Derrick.

After I had Derrick, I didn't pay the rent, and I got evicted from the apartment. They made us go down to the Housing Authority, and they told me they were putting me in Bracken Field in West Hill. I said, "Where the hell is it?" I'd never heard of it. But I knew what the hell, I had no choice, I had to do it. So hell, fine, on the first of September we moved in.

Bracken Field. What a place! See, like where all the time I was growing up, of course, everybody's poor. But everybody owned their own land, their own house, their own farm, grew their own food, caught their own fish, you know, this kind of thing, so you really don't need a whole lot of cash. The house I grew up in was kind of rackety, cold running water. We had electricity. Some of the people didn't. We had an old wood stove, and like in the winter the house was colder than hell. But the housing situation is different than people that grew up in the city. Because I really cannot get myself to accept the whole business—the same damn thing which Senator Muskie said, which they wouldn't put into Time Magazine, because it had sexual overtones—when people live on top of people, they begin to eat each other up. In the housing project that's just what they do. These people here are cutting these people here's throats.

You live there, and you can see it. It's a whole mental thing about living in a housing project. My sleeping habits and my eating habits are the ones I grew up with and they're different than the people that grew up in the city. I think black people have their own particular habits anyway. I like to go to bed at eight thirty or nine o'clock at night, and I like to get up at four or five in the morning. I like to get up in the morning, wash the kitchen floor, do my laundry and hang it outdoors and do all my work in the morning. Over here in the project, people are just going to bed! In the warm weather they're just going to bed at three or four o'clock in the morning when it starts to get daylight, and they sleep all day. And about four in the afternoon, they start coming out. When you come to work in the morning, most of the kids you see out are white kids, the black kids come out later. It's the way they live—they're nocturnal people. I'm not. So shoot, I go to bed and try to sleep.

Shoot, they're out there dancing in the street, dancing upstairs overhead with real loud music which I can't stand either. And the kids raising hell in the hallway. It's the middle of my night. It's the middle of their day. All this just drives me up a wall. I really can't stand it, and anyway I can't stand noise. I can't stand traffic noise. I can't stand sirens going, and in the project two or three times a night the fire engines are coming. And, of course, the police are always banging around when you don't need them, and when you need them they're not there. People . . . like the first night I moved . . . the first night I stayed in the project, of course, I couldn't sleep too good anyways. And this lady yelling and she's running down Ford Street. "I love you . . . I don't want you to leave . . . I want you to be my man forever." She's carrying on like this, and she didn't hardly have any clothes on. Here's this man trudging down the road, and she's hanging after him, telling him she needs him. You'd think to Christ somebody was putting on a theatre show or something. This kind of stuff just goes on. Then you hear . . . "I'm going to slit your throat." "Don't touch me . . . don't." I mean the stuff that goes on . . . smashing bottles, and roaches . . . and Jesus . . . I mean the whole thing just gets on your nerves. You're worrying about one damn thing after another. Like the incinerator's in the hallway. I like to empty my trash right after a meal, get rid of it right away. So then, the nuns moved in, and one of them got attacked in the hallway six o'clock at night. I didn't even dare take my trash out and empty it in the incinerator.

When I went on welfare, I met Trudy, and I started working with her to organize people on welfare. At that time people were ashamed to say they was on welfare . . . it was a big shame thing, much worse than it is today. Trudy is a very good organizer, smart as hell. She can psych people out, and she's not scared of anybody, whereas I was still at that time kind of shy. People who were my own thing I could get along with very well. People in police uniforms, people who were social workers, I was still scared of.

But when I moved into Bracken Field, I stopped working with

Trudy so much, because I didn't have time to go down there. So then I started working as a neighborhood worker out of the CAP agency in West Hill. It was a Title 5 Program. Welfare let me work twenty hours a week, and they paid me twenty-seven dollars and fifty cents every two weeks for it, plus they paid my baby-sitter. By this time Danny was driving me crazy, being with him every day all day long was getting to be too much. An old lady from Vermont that I knew, and who reminded me of my grandmother, agreed to come to my house three days a week to take care of the boys. So I went to work and got to know all the people who were running CAP in West Hill—Tom Leaner, Ned Handler, Andy Fitch.

Ned was putting out a good newsletter, but he and Fitch didn't get along because they had different ideas, and Ned's a strong personality. At the same time I was working with Ned going into people's homes that the social workers said were having difficulties. I ran into some what you call multi-problem families over there, especially in those old rickety wooden buildings near the railroad tracks that are being torn down now.

It makes you wonder about people, honest to God. This girl had four kids, one that was just little, teeny. She was Irish, married to a Cuban guy, and she had this other Cuban guy she was living with who was a pimp. She was a prostitute and all those little babies. The house was filthy . . . filthy rotten. One day I went over to her house, her little girl was two years old then, and she was just burned. We rushed her into hospital. They questioned the mother about child abuse, and the mother says that she sent the little girl to take a bath, and she ran the water too hot and jumped in and got burned! While that little girl was in the hospital the little baby drank some brown furniture polish. The mother said the baby was crawling on the floor and found it and drank it. They said the baby couldn't possibly lift it up to drink it. The mother must have rammed it down his throat.

I don't believe in state authorities or anybody else coming in and telling you how to run your house, or how to take care of your kids . . . I'm against that. I'm against taking kids away from mothers, but damn, sometimes those babies have to be protected too. Because some of these mothers are not in a mental state at certain times to take care of as many problems as three or four kids represent. You get yourself in a bad situation . . . you don't know where the hell to turn, and you've got a bad man hanging around telling you bad things to do. It's your kids are going to be suffering. Something's got to be done about that.

I was going into different houses and trying to work with the mothers where they felt that somebody that's on welfare themselves and in a bad situation themselves has a better way of getting along with somebody else in a bad situation than a social worker. That's true in most cases I think, but, then again, somebody such as myself can only go a certain path. In some of these cases, you have to know a doctor so you can call him up and say, "Look doctor, I'm sorry as hell, I know you're busy, but can you get over here right now to this house and try to do something." Because sometimes you need a doctor in there, not a social worker. Sometimes you need the police in there.

I gained some experience working there. Sometimes I'd take Danny and Derrick to the CAP office with me. Ned was having a biff with Mrs. Morton who had the Day Care Center in Bracken Field. All black kids and white teachers. Mrs. Morton who's black, is whiter than half the white teachers. Ned thought they could put some black pictures on the walls and use a little imagination. I've been carrying on the same biff with Mrs. Morton for the last three years, and the school has changed. We've got four parents on the Board now, and last summer we had three parents hired as teachers for the summer camp.

So I worked under Title 5 at the CAP. Okay, but welfare don't give you enough money to live on. Like I don't waste money, but they don't give you enough for food. *My* kids are not drinking skimmed milk. I don't give a damn if it goes up to a dollar a half gallon, I'm going to buy milk. I buy three half gallons a day. Danny drinks a whole lot of milk. If he wants Bosco in his milk, I'm going to put Bosco in his milk. I buy fresh vegetables. They had peas in the pod the other day . . . a little thing . . . *a dollar* at the supermarket. I eat them raw, that's the only way I like them. And shoot, if the kids were up home, they'd be out in the garden stealing them in the summertime, chewing on them and digging up carrots and eating them. When Derrick's a bit older, I'll send them up home for a month. I want them to get to know Grammie. She's got a lot to offer because she loves little kids.

I kept on Title 5 till it dissolved and became part of the Work Incentive Program and I went on that. But they cut us down from twenty-seven dollars and fifty cents every two weeks to fifteen dollars every two weeks. This is progress via welfare. Meanwhile I was meeting people in the area and we started having meetings to try to set up our own day care center. We've just heard that Model Cities is giving us money for renovations. Course the person in charge of Model Cities don't know anything. He's in a powerful position and not capable of handling it. This is part of the system's way of getting people fed up. That's why they put Drake to head the poverty program in the early days. They know if they put a jackass up there, that all the people were going to be fed up with the program.

Anyhow we got some foundation money, and we set up two courses—Childhood Growth and Development and Early Childhood Curriculum, to get us more familiar and give us books to read and the direction to learn more. Sixteen of us took courses two days a week, and the other three days went to observe at different day care centers. The foundation money paid the transportation money, babysitting money, thirty-six dollars a week for the sixteen people that took the courses for three months.

But see, doctor, once you start getting involved in one thing, then that carries on to something else. I didn't have any intentions whatsoever of getting involved in the Health Advisory Group. I was involved in the Modernization Committee. I was involved in the nursery school in Bracken Field trying to organize the parents. One thing I'll say good about the nursery school—they have excellent social workers trained specifically in dealing with young children and mothers. There was always a long waiting list for the school, but the children were chosen because of a particular need of a particular family. Chosen because of the child and the mother. Now the whole emphasis has changed. To get a child into nursery school, the mother has to work. Or be on the Work Incentive Program. Now that's bullshit.

I was on the Modernization Committee from the beginning because I was chairman of the rat and roach committee, which I'd set up myself because I was dealing with some rats over at the Nursery School. I still haven't dealt with that problem successfully. And I was also working with senior citizens. Well Lily Finn was with the Health Advisory group and was real excited about it. I was real happy inside myself that Lily found something she could get involved in with other people. It was very therapeutic, and I was sad when she moved out of the project because I felt it was a step down for her. She kept telling me to come . . . come . . . . But I had a thing about the Clinic. Derrick used to stop breathing. He'd turn blue and collapse and stop breathing. The first time it happened I went out of my mind. Well the doctors at the Health Center told me it was temper tantrums and he'd be okay. I got mad at the Clinic. I got mad at East Childrens Hospital. I went to Tate, and they did a complete workup and said he was all right. I felt much better.

So I had a bad thing against the Health Center. But I had known you, and you were a real positive piece of propaganda for the Clinic, I mean being there and everything. I decided the best way to find out about the Clinic was to get involved in it. So I took Lily's advice, and one day when they were discussing something I was really interested in I came. After I came to the first meeting, I really started coming.

I don't believe that any professional—I don't care how long he's gone to school—I really don't think they can get any course which is really going to change their basic attitude towards dealing with poor people. Most people do not like poor people, and if they end up dealing with poor people that underlying feeling is very evident, although they try to keep it covered up. It comes out. And poor people are very, very sensitive and pick these things up. Certain people can come right in, and they fit right in fine. And certain people . . . that thing isn't there, whatever it is. So you end up having to deal with this kind of people that you don't like to deal with, like most of the people in the Housing Authority. Now how do you deal with them as a community group? How do you deal with these professionals effectively to get changes that you want to see made? To do it it's essential for the Health Committee to know how much involved politics are with everything . . . with running the Health Center, and the Housing Authority, running the Department of Community Affairs, running who gets into low-income housing and who doesn't. Who gets sewerage and who doesn't. Who gets the street cleaned and who doesn't.

The Health Advisory Committee has to have training. That's positive, they have to. Now, see, like certain people in the Committee may already be pretty aware, but other members may not be aware at all, and if you're not aware at all then you tend to say well politics doesn't have nothing to do with it. But like in the job I'm

working at now, in the New Careers part that I'm in, they feel that
it's very essential that we, if we're going to be community or-
ganizers, get to understand the whole process of how to file a bill
. . . which bills get through and which ones don't . . . and what
state representatives vote for it and which ones don't vote for it
. . . how come . . . who is pressuring who to get it done . . . right
on up to the President . Which is politics, which is a hell of a boring
subject.

But you have to know that because you can bang your head
against a damn wall, and it's not going to change anything. You really have to know all that stuff. And so for a group of volunteer
community people who have all their own kids, all their own every
day stuff they have to take care of, to volunteer their time to come
in to these meetings to try to get something done; to also try to
enlarge upon their knowledge to be more effective, it takes time
and it's going to take money. And the people don't have very much
time and nobody has any money. There has to be money involved
in there somewhere. I really, really don't like the idea of paying
people to go to meetings, but it seems to be the most effective way.
Because the people need the money.

I, personally, think it would be better, say, once a year everybody that has been active in the thing through the year get a flat
amount. Get a check in the mail for a flat amount of money. Along
with a letter stating, "We appreciate your activities" and that kind
of thing. I don't know where the money would come from. I don't
think it should be from the Health Center. Because then there
would be resentment among some of the staff. I feel it should come
from the Department of Health, Education and Welfare. That's
what I think because it's health, and it's education and it's welfare.

The first time I went to a Health Committee meeting I said,
"This group is really together." I was getting disillusioned with the
CAP agency because they weren't doing anything. So then I really
started going to the meetings, and I really got involved in it.

Of course I don't get along with all the Health Center staff. I
don't get along with Mrs. Lally at all. You know she takes the kids,
who are supposed to be emotionally disturbed, in her special class.
She's from Tennessee, and she's white, white, white. She don't
know a damn thing about kids either. She doesn't really understand. You know Danny's in Mrs. Lally's group. Danny called
Mrs. Lally "whitey," so Mrs. Lally came back to me, and she said

I must have told Danny to call her that name because she knew
Danny was only four years old, and he isn't able to distinguish a
white person from a black person at his age. And I said, "Jumping
Christ, you're a child specialist or something, and you think that he
knows the difference between blue, purple and red and orange, and
you think he don't know the difference between a black person and
a white person? With a black father that he's very close to and a
white mother? For Christ sake . . . living in the project. Are you
serious? Watching the news? You think he don't know the difference? What's wrong with you?" And see, I threw up my hands.
Then I was thinking about it afterwards. I said, "Well maybe Mrs.
L. was trying to find out what kind of a reaction I was going to
have. Maybe that's why she did it. Or maybe she just for real didn't
think Danny knew the difference between white people and black
people." Well you see why she's not able to help these kind of
children. Anyhow I was getting teed off—why the hell Mrs. Lally
had the right to say that my chile or anybody else's was emotionally disturbed when Dr. Dick was telling me that he wasn't, but
he was spoiled rotten.

I think the Health Clinic could take a much more effective role
in trying to get the whole development upgraded. I think they definitely could. If the community people do something, the code enforcement people won't pay any attention to the community people. If the Health Clinic tries to push something, it does. Why the
hell don't the Health Center force the code enforcement people to
do something about these elevators around here. Just as one example, the damn elevators.

Ideally all the organizations in the project could work
together, but they're not going to. No. You've got Joseph Eaton.
He's sharp, but there's a teeny weeny element there missing. I
never figured out Joseph Eaton. Like he decided that what this development needed was inter-agency meetings. And he sent out all
these nice letters to the heads of all the agencies to come to the
Health Center, and he would chair it to figure out what each group
was doing, and what they were supposed to be doing, and what
they could do together to get something done. Well of course this
was the same thing that Reverend Farmer tried. And that didn't
turn out very effectively either. Well everybody came to that meeting. People from the Nursery School, Housing, CAP, Modernization, Tenant Management, Active Mothers . . . there was just or-

ganizations all over the place. Of course, they did a whole lot of talking and decided to set up sub-committees and to get together again the next week. They had a few meetings, and the last one I showed up at they were discussing why more people don't come. Joseph Eaton wasn't there . . . he hadn't showed up for the last three meetings. It's comical. But, well, it's damn discouraging.

I don't know hardly anybody that lives in that project that I could really say has got their two feet on the ground as to who they are, or where they're from, or where they're going. *I'm* not in that situation, and maybe, therefore, I don't think anybody else is, but I really don't think so. Part of the experience of being poor, you know, you just say, "What the hell . . . what the hell." I mean that's a good attitude to have part of the time and part of the time it isn't . . . "what the hell . . . what the hell." You can get to a point where you say, "What the hell . . . there's garbage all over the place . . . what the hell." See, you shouldn't get to that point because that's going too far. But you have to have that attitude about some things.

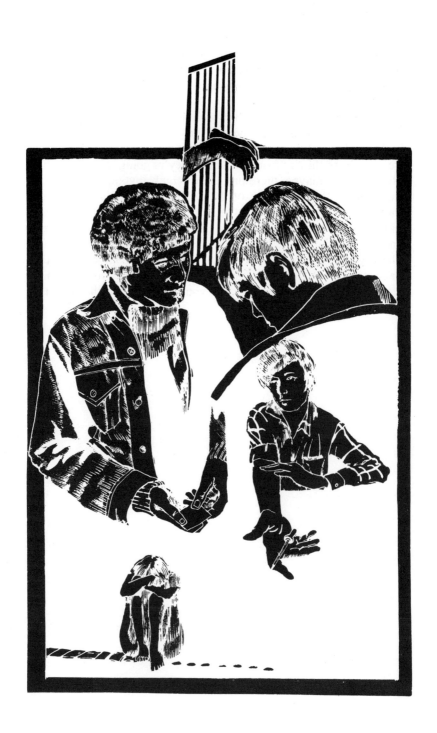

Chapter II

Drug Unit

Cecil — Junkie or Ex-Addict?
The Struggle Against Drugs

At seventeen, after two years in the Army, Cecil married his girlfriend who had already borne his daughter. Cecil's first contact with marijuana and heroin was during this period of Army service.

Cecil drifted from one job to another. While still living with his wife, he impregnated another woman who left him after having a criminal abortion. At this time his wife also left him, and, in despair and anger, he began first to snort heroin regularly and then to inject it. For a year and a half he supported himself and his habit by shoplifting, but was finally caught and jailed. From then on he kept returning to jail for shoplifting. All told he served eight years.

When we met Cecil, he was being treated in the Drug Addiction Unit of the State Psychiatric Hospital. He was in an experimental program which used group therapy and confrontation techniques and had been off heroin six months. A group of residents in the housing project had set up a Drug Committee and a Drug Unit with the help and medical back-up service of our staff. The committee invited Cecil and another ex-addict, Mario, to work in the Drug Unit.

I learned a lot in prison. There I started to really utilize the time and do something constructive. I read. I did a lot of art work. I played sports. I stayed out of trouble. I was never locked up like guys are for fighting or drugs. People don't believe that you can get just as much drugs in jails as you can in the street. I kicked all my habits in jail, you know, except for the one I kicked at East State (heroin). They have screws that are money hungry that will bring these drugs in for the guys. One guy was getting whiskey, and they charged him ten dollars for a pint of whiskey. The guys would pool their money and get the whiskey.

Yes, it's true that I went off drugs in jail and back on drugs out of jail. What I see now, I didn't see until I started working in the Drug Unit of the Health Center, helping other people get off drugs. I didn't see it until I started doing this job here and dealing with feelings in the groups. I stayed up nights trying to figure out why a guy will be off drugs, and swear to all the gods that this is the last time and mean it. I could never understand it before, but after working with the kids for a few months, now I do. The reason is simple . . . you're afraid.

Afraid of outside . . . the world . . . people . . . responsibilities. For instance, the average kid now that's doing drugs is a drop-out from school, right? The majority of these guys hasn't prepared themselves for nothing, you know, as far as a job is concerned, and yet people are saying, even stronger now than when I was coming up, "You're not going to even be able to push brooms because like, man, they got machines now to do all that." They show you pictures, and you go to the movies; where they used to have a porter, or manpower, they got a machine to do these things. You turn around if you've got anything on the ball and look at things like the railroads . . . that's one of the most pitiful things in the world to me right now. So all these things scare you, and you're out here and you know what's waiting for you . . . nothing but destruction.

You're likely to go back into the world and do the same things that you went to jail for, because if you look at it the way it really is, you haven't prepared yourself for nothing . . . you don't know anything to do. The only thing you have going for you, most black people (I don't know about the white kids) is construction . . . hard, back-breaking . . . but the guy that picks up the boards and rolls the wheelbarrow can make two and one-half dollars an hour, and with overtime can take home a nice pay to his wife, or his mother or wherever he's living, right?

But now, who do I know that can get me the job? Well, I know Jim Jones, but Jim Jones will want to know can he trust you because Jim Jones done bought some of the hot goods that you used to have so Jim Jones knows that you are not reliable . . . that you're not going to be able to work . . . that you're going to use dope. So what do you do? You got to come right back where you came from—stealing. And when you steal, you get right back in with the dope because all the frustrations, the uptightness, insecure feelings and everything is wrapped up right there waiting for you, and you know it's there, and that's why you're scared.

That's why when you're putting on your clothes that last day, that's when you tell yourself, "Man, can I make it this time, will I make it this time? Can't stay in the house every day, 'cause you know, you get tired of that, and from the time you walk out the door, until you stick that spike in your arm, you're scared . . . petrified. This is why as soon as the guy gets off the bus or the train—if he saved any money—he goes, and he starts making preparations to go back to jail where he's safe.

He goes to my house—he's been away six or seven months, and he don't know how hot my house is, whether they're watching it or not—he goes with some friends that he met in the street. "Who got it?" "Cecil got it." "Well, we'll go to Cecil's house." Or he might ask, "Is it cool there?" The guy he asks hasn't got money but he knows you got money . . . he might want that money . . . so he says, "Oh, yeah, it's cool." Cops probably hanging out of the ceiling light fixture, but that's the lie he's going to tell you because he wants that fix, so you go. Sometimes guys will be out a matter of hours, and they're on their way back. You take that shot, and then you go home. You don't have to listen to the beefs because you're high; if your wife is really slack and the house is filthy, you don't have to look at it; you don't have to look at your Mom still working when she should be retired; you don't have to look at the little dirty kids that don't even have a chance, and they're running and laughing and playing, and you're saying to yourself, "Man, I wonder what he's going to be like . . . I wonder what she's going to be like?"

And you look at the people that are in positions to help to do something about this thing and they're playing games, too. They don't care about those kids, they don't care about me, they don't care about anybody, but they tell people that they care. The guy that really needs the help got to look at that. You've got to see that, and, man, how am I going to make it, and I got this fear on me. So that's why a guy needs drugs when he comes out.

Ex-Addict Mario —
One Mother But Seven Fathers

When Cecil started working in the Health Center Drug Unit, he introduced Mario to us and suggested that he join the staff of the Drug Unit. Mario was the child of his mother's first marriage—his father died when he was three years old. His mother had seven marriages in all. He had an unhappy childhood fighting with his stepfathers, siblings and peers and was unable to communicate with his mother. White, of Swiss-Italian background, he grew up in a household prejudiced against blacks.

He, himself, married and divorced three times and has three children whom he has not seen in seven years. An intelligent, articulate but immature and undereducated youth, he turned his talents to safe-breaking and robbed twenty-two safes before he was caught and jailed.

I had my first taste of heroin in prison. I had smoked marijuana for about ten years before that, but there wasn't any dependence on it. I wasn't using it to cop out. When I got in prison, all of a sudden I had to deal with the fact that I had failed in three marriages. I had to deal with the fact that I wasn't destined for any of the great things that I had predestined myself for.

I was in jail for seventeen months, and I came out a cold-blooded dope addict. Matter of fact when I came out the Federal Pen, I was high. After I was released from jail, I went to live in the East State (Mental Hospital) Half-way House. I went through the program there, got a job, and got myself together. I was secretary to the credit union at the Half-way House. I was trying to make it back; so I decided to go back to school. I went back to school, and first thing I got jammed! I just blew that whole thing. I didn't have any study habits, and it was difficult to grasp concepts. The only real education I had was the seventeen months in the penitentiary. I had books. I wanted to know all kinds of abstractions because I thought there's something better than where I'm at, and I have to grasp the basic concepts first before I can get that together and translate it to where I am. I was reading philosophy in prison, and seeing how Thomas Mann differed from Kierkegaard or from Sartre. That was my great self-education period. I really learned a lot, but I didn't know how to apply it, because practically speaking I had been down so long I didn't know how to get up.

I got married the third time four months after I got out of jail. A young teacher in East City . . . very pretty . . . intelligent . . . couldn't ask for a better wife. But a wife wasn't what I wanted. I wanted somebody to keep the loneliness away and to keep this parole thing off my back. I was using dope, but my wife didn't know. She suspected something was wrong, but she couldn't put her finger on it.

But she did have experience with a junkie . . . with me . . . she saved my life. I was working and making a lot of money at that time, bringing home about two hundred and twenty dollars a week, and doing well. Plus, I was selling dope on the side to support my habit.

But then my whole world just went up; I couldn't deal with it anymore, and I O.D.'d . . . overdosed . . . in fact I think I cooked up ten bags of dope at one time. I guess I was trying to kill myself, but really wasn't consciously aware of what I was trying to do. So I got off . . . I didn't really pass out . . . it was just a very heavy nod, but I was very aware of what was going on around me. The sensation was like every cell in my body was dying . . . right from the tip of my toes. I had the feeling it was right up to my chest. When it got up to my chest it felt like breathing was very, very hard.

I wasn't panicked, but I wanted to say, "Help me." I felt like I was dying. My wife came in . . . from work . . . she opened the bathroom door and said, "Hey, what's going on?" I was lying there with this thing sticking out of my leg. When she realized what it was, she got a saline solution, some salt and some orange stuff, and injected me with it. She had had some nurse training. She got me up and walking around, and I started coming around. I went into the hospital the next day . . . East State Hospital because I saw what happened. I just saw my whole thing going, my life . . . this whole chaotic thing . . . I stop and look back, and I can't account for ten years of my life.

I was in the hospital about three months and a few days; it was a turning point in my life. Okay, I got out of East State, and I saw that the world wasn't really an oyster. Nobody was going to give me anything; anything I got I was going to have to get myself by my own efforts. I was prepared to deal with it.

In the meantime, at East State there'd been a profound change in people's attitudes, and in my own demeanor. They asked me, "Hey, would you be interested in working here at State?" "Gee,

would I really?'' So they kind of let me run groups. I was doing
very well. Then of course, this drug unit came up here at the Health
Center.

I had taken over Cecil's group at times at State because Cecil
was away most of the time. One day he asked me to come to the
Health Center with him. I went up there and wow—I couldn't
believe it; it's just incredible, the attitude that some of these people
had about drugs. As time went on, I decided to work in the Drug
Unit. I can relate to black people as well as I can relate to white
people, and I'm certainly educated to the street level idiom
because of my dope experience, and because of experience with
black people.

When I was young, I used to fight black people all the time. I
was one of the most prejudiced people in the world when I was
about thirteen or fourteen, though I never saw a black person until
I went to school. I'm Swiss-Italian, but I didn't live in an Italian environment. I was brought up in a very prejudiced household. There
wasn't very much understanding of the black thing at all. It was accepted that black people were stupid, and, ''I'm not going to have
any niggers in my house.''

All this conditioning had made me hate, without really knowing what hate was or why I hated. Finally we got this kid in junior
high school, the only black kid in the school. I wonder what the hell
he felt like. I started digging myself . . . looking at myself and saying, ''It's strange, this kid is black, and he really isn't stupid, this
kid's kind of smart, at least as smart as I am.'' I was a straight A
student when I was in high school, right on through. Never had any
problems in school, in terms of grades. I always had problems with
my attitude. I had a very bad attitude towards authority, and I was
really miserable. I was very difficult to get along with.

I used to talk to this black kid. I talked about his blackness,
and then he'd talk about it. He was conservative actually. His
father was a Lt. Colonel in the Army, and he was kind of very well
off for a black person, living in a white community, and oh man, the
tokenism that used to go on was really sickening. He's probably a
dope addict himself now. But anyway, he liked me, and I got
somewhat close to him. I became involved with him, and when I
left home I felt myself for some reason being drawn toward black
people.

I went into the Service. My best friend was black—Ned Jefferson from L.A.—the only kid in the unit from L.A. We got along . . . a great big monstrous fellow—one of the biggest black guys I ever saw. He went to basic training with me, and we stuck together through the whole thing like brothers . . . buddies.

Ned was very articulate and very smart. We just got along real well, and I seemed to be hanging out with black people more and more. As a matter of fact that's where I was introduced to mari-juana . . . this cat and I smoking reefer together . . . hash. I was a little man—the shortest guy in the whole outfit.

Right after that I got married to a Corsican, an Algerian girl from Paris. She was a Corps de Ballet teacher, also a folk-singer, very beautiful, very bright, intelligent, vivacious. Needless to say, we didn't get along. She was just as demanding as I was for affec-tion. I couldn't really give to her, and she couldn't give to me, but we were very much in love at the same time. We had a son. But I lost out in that marriage, and, in about a year and a half, I came back on the rebound and got married again. My second marriage was a consequence of my first failure. The third failure was the re-sult of the second failure. Things never got any better.

I sought help for a while when I was in the penitentiary, yeah, I was very familiar with the department of medicine. But the fellow I was seeing couldn't reach me. I would just sit there for two hours, and when the time was up, I'd pay and I'd split. I saw psychiatry was not the answer to my problem. In fact, the only person that could help me was myself, but I didn't know how to do it. And that's what I got over at State (Mental Hospital). I found out how to do it, how to handle things and how to love people.

I started seeing myself in other people. I started seeing I wasn't the only one in the world who'd suffered; I wasn't the only one who had had failed marriages; I wasn't the only one who'd been in prison; I wasn't the only one who didn't have any father; I wasn't the only one that still loved his mother but was also mad at her for giving him such a screwed up life. I was big enough to un-derstand it finally.

I must have cried for four or five hours when I was in the group psychiatry session—the marathon went on for twelve hours, and dealt with me for about four hours out of that. When I finished with this marathon, everybody in the whole room was crying, not *for* me but *with* me 'cause I'd gone through this kind of hassle. It was the most beautiful, enlightening experience I've ever had in my life. At the end of the marathon I thought, "Well, I am basically a good person; I have a lot of things to give people," and after that I started building up faith and trust in myself. So like I said, I decided to work in the Health Center Drug Unit.

I went to live in Bracken Field, joined the club across the street with the youngsters, talked to the kids, became involved in the West Hill organization for health and eventually became involved in other things that were happening in the area. I had my finger on the pulse of things. I knew what was going on, I was interested in the community, and I was really getting things done. Like going out on a speaking engagement and rapping with all those people that were really interested in what was happening, or doing something very dynamic, like going on TV with a group to show people that we were doing things, getting something together. There's a strange necessity for me to do that kind of thing. It's very productive, and it keeps me with that sense of fulfillment. I'm always innovating on ways to be more creative—to bring out more in the group. People become fascinating when they get in the group, and they start participating. I've really noted a lot of things that aren't in psych books.

If you've been there yourself, you have an inside track from a practical point of view, from actual living. By the same token you can identify with all strata of society, no matter what level. My concern is with the parts that we're forgetting, like for instance the black ghetto and the white ghetto also. They really hassle me. The Police Department bothers me too because there's police brutality. I'm currently involved as a witness in a case of police brutality where a cop came down and started beating on a kid.

I see my job working in the Drug Clinic as a temporary thing. When a black man comes out of that particular community into my group and I train him and make sure he can handle my job, he can take my place. I see that not only with the Drug Unit; I see it in all of Bracken Field. I see that with the Clinic and with various other social agencies that are in there. I really see black people running those kinds of things. It's theirs; it's in their particular area where they live. I don't see that we have to import all the professionals.

Living in the housing project? I was very depressed most of the time because I saw the kids playing out there with nothing better to do than break windows, and throw rocks at each other, and kind of wallow in their own mire, their own helplessness. There's all these outside elements pushing in which kind of creates an invisible wall around there; you don't know exactly where the wall is, but it's there, and within that wall there's a lot of pressure because these people can't get out from inside. Bracken Field, you know, should be destroyed.

But you have to take into consideration, what's happening there . . . why the kids go in the hallway and urinate . . . why they bust all the windows, break all the lights . . . what are they telling you? They're telling you they don't like the place . . . they're telling you they don't have anything constructive to do. They're telling you, "You're not giving us anything . . . you're not giving us our own place." They're telling the CAP not just the Health Center, "You're saying you want to help us, but man, all we see are white faces coming into our place." Okay. I hear that. Okay, now what is it that's so hopeless about living in this place, because like I ask you guys, what is it about this place that you really hate? Fact is, you don't know what you hate, but you see people driving better cars, or you see pictures of people doing better things on TV. You know there's something better than exists over the hill or around the corner because you've either seen it, or heard about it or some damn thing, but you don't have it, and the chances are that you aren't going to have it, and within that, boy, there's a lot of futility.

The way I'd deal with the drug problem is to approach all the social agencies and schools, and probably the churches, any organization that's on a community level, even the Neighborhood Employment Office, welfare agencies and so on. I'd present them with an educational preventive program that would consist of using ex-addicts or addicts, along with maybe audio-visual aids. Or maybe I'd just use the kids themselves—articulate kids that can convey feeling to these people, explaining what the dangers are, what's happening with drugs, what goes on—not using any scare tactics but on a very practical level showing them where it's really at, what's happening, what it can lead to. Kids can answer questions that adults just can't answer. Whether such programs inspire curiosity or not, that's irrelevant; kids are curious to begin with, and if they want to experiment, they're going to experiment anyway, but at least let them know what the possibilities of their experimentation are; the possibility that they can kill themselves by taking heroin; the possibility that if you smoke reefer you might have a psychotic reaction to it, and what's happening with speed and amphetamines; what the chances are of hurting yourself. It would be good to explain, and have people that are very professional in that, explain these things to kids. And make it a regular course in high school.

Some of the kids are kind of lost in this black thing. This is what one kid told me in the group. "A white man's got no business in this group; a black man should be handling it." I turned around and said, "Well, here you are, man. Handle it, it's your job, you handle it. Show me that you can do a better job than I can. Prove it to me and you can have my job." He couldn't deal with that—didn't know what the hell to do with it. So then I said, "Well, okay, you can't deal with it, can you man? So stay the hell out of my business; don't put me down unless you can handle it." And the kid . . . it was all he could do to restrain himself . . . he wanted to punch me out. I told him, "You get hostile towards me for something I'm doing. I worked without money for many months; I don't have to live in this slum, man, but I live in it. I choose to live in it because I want to know what's happening. It's cats like you that are making the slums. You as an individual. Here you are, a super-junkie taking dope, and you're going to try and tell me what the hell I'm doing. At least I'm doing something in the community. You haven't contributed a damn thing other than take dope or sell dope. Where you should really be, man, is out there trying to stop that action, if you really care about yourself. Apparently you don't care about yourself, you're still using dope, and you haven't taken advantage of the hospital." For the most part, the kids respect an opinion from me because I'm giving it to them as straight as I possibly can.

You want them to care about themselves . . . to care about what's going to happen tomorrow . . . to care about this whole situation . . . black-white society—all part of the big picture. You also have to see that there really are rats and cockroaches living in Bracken Field. You have to know, too, that you've got limitations, and you can't do it all yourself. Just for the moment, I have to live with the establishment, but I also have to live with this gross tragedy, the fact that Bracken Field exists. We have to live with that, but what can we best do to effect change within that community? How do we deal with the junkie? How do we deal with the apathy in terms of maintenance? How do we deal with CAP— what's the best situation for a movement like CAP within this whole spectrum of ideas? All these things have to be taken into consideration. It's tremendously hard.

I think that the Health Center has in several ways contributed to helping the community, and the junkies. Oh, wow—meanwhile it's helped also in a criminal way. It's been ripped off, been broken into so many times, people have stolen so much out of it, I guess it has certainly helped the hoodlum element! One of the biggest things, I think, is the fact that the people who are working in the Health Center, whether they're white or black, are very sincerely and truly motivated for the most part. All the chicks in there . . . really there's no duality in their motivations. Most of the people there are very happy, trying to get something together, really dedicated people. Just talking to people they have bettered relationships in the community; just by going out and and rapping and being concerned they have improved relationships immensely. Without the Health Center right now, I feel there would be a lot of pressure manifested in terms of a very noisy war. Without the Drug Unit, most of the junkies out there would be hitting each other over the head and killing each other. Without the Health Center, West Hill would be in serious trouble. The Health Center has become very active and very interested in participating in all the programs in Bracken Field. It helps very much just from the perspective of caring.

Basically, I think for the most part people want to get along. I think there's a lot of people who've got their particular hangups, and black people are just as prejudiced as white people. We're demonstrating that we can work together because we've got black people incorporated into the Health Center that have very responsible positions. There's a lot going on with black people that live in the community and that's a fact. People like Mabel Straley who are super, super-human. She really does a lot. Yeah, she just knocks me out. I heard her come out and say, "Well, my own son is a dope addict, and I have to try and deal with that."

I learned at State, that there's more to life than dying. Once I went as far as to write my own epitaph without even realizing it. I wrote a poem:

> Not a cross to mark the spot
> Where I lay in eternal sleep
> But instead a gambler's coin
> For it was by a flip and toss
> That I lost the game of life or death.

I was saying I took a chance—I wrote this while I was using dope—
and I lost, and so for mankind, I really didn't count.

I tell you, I could never in a million years sit behind a desk.
There's too much need for communication. I have to be in the
center somewhere, dealing within that, even if it's just an emotional nucleus. I have to be there to check it and feel its vibrations,
and feel the dynamics of it, be a part of it, because that's basically
where my feelings are. I still get high, but the kind of high that I get
is of the spirit. For the first time I can appreciate what it's like to be
in love with a person. For the first time I can appreciate what it's
like to grieve when a person's lost.

I really feel that what I told a group of residents at East
Children's Hospital last month sums up the way I see things now.
"There are certain experiences that I've had that you haven't had
as a doctor. You're there to treat something you know; you've
learned to treat an illness. You can't prevent the illness from coming on unless you know where the heck it's at. I know where the illness comes from, because I have a pretty good idea of where I'm
at, who I am, and where I'm going, and I'm not unmindful of
anybody else, but I have an inside track, a unique perspective of
myself, and I consider myself as much of a professional as you."

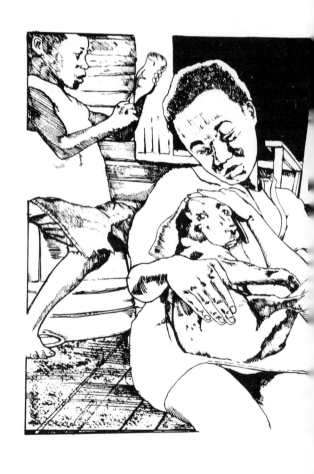

Chapter III

Opinion Leaders

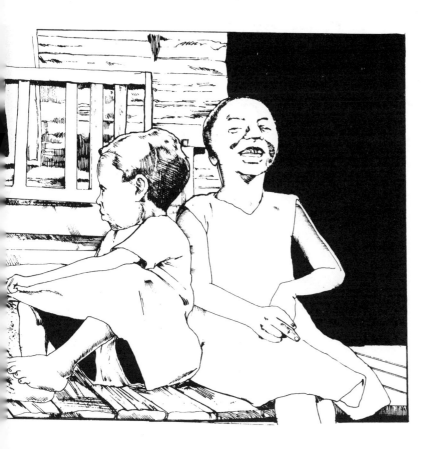

Robert Prescott —
From State Ward to Housing Manager

Robert Prescott, a highly respected community leader who became Manager of Bracken Field Housing Project a year after I left the Health Center, is the father of twelve children all of whom he is determined will receive college educations. He has an intense interest in furthering educational opportunities, particularly for blacks.

Both Robert's parents died in his infancy. The children were separated from each other and placed in foster homes as wards of the State. Until the age of sixteen when by sheer chance he met his oldest brother, Robert did not know that his parents had died—he thought he had been abandoned. His earliest experiences in foster homes were horrifying, though at five he was placed with a loving family with whom he remained until he was reunited with his own family. The neighborhood school he attended was almost completely white and, as he recalls, far above his income level. As a result he suffered from discrimination and acute embarrassment throughout his school career. After only two years of high school, he became a laborer in a shipyard before going into the Armed Services.

It was the kind of things that happened to me all my life that led me towards trying to work towards a better life for black people. Let's take it back to when I was going to school. I had told the guidance counsellor that I would like to be an engineer on a railroad, operating the big locomotive. I was told that there's no job for Negroes as engineers on the railroad. If you're smart enough and work hard enough, maybe you could be a fireman on the locomotive. I played football and hockey professionally. The coach told me to look for something else . . . a boxer maybe . . . a musician . . . a tap dancer. Hockey wasn't ready to accept Negroes then.

I was in constant trouble at school, fighting white kids who called me names. The principal—I hated her guts—would say to me, "Well, Robert, I don't know what I'm going to do to make you realize that sticks and stones may break your bones, but names should never hurt you." I could tell you many other things, but that's the kind of things I mean.

The first thing I did in the community interest was to join the

AmVets, a black organization of Army Veterans. I'm still a member. I became their Assistant Recreational Officer and worked with the teenagers. I got to know Dean Roke pretty well through the AmVets. He was running in a second term try for Representative from Ward Twelve in East City, and I started doing some campaigning for him. The more I worked for Dean the more I found out how much prejudice there was, hidden behind closed doors. I found out about forces working hard to keep a black man from getting into public office. We ran into things where so-called outstanding white citizens of Old Town (that was the Jewish element then) actually paid through the nose to have other black people run against Dean, just to chop up the black vote. We really didn't have enough black votes anyway at that time for Dean to win— compared to the white people living in Old Town at that time we were still outnumbered. When we started clashing with certain elements of the power structure, I began to learn many things. I learned how they fine-talk out of one side of their face, and how they stay up all hours of the night to block you from achieving what you might want to do.

I was living in Old Town at the time and I was married. I remember we had a big fight over on Blue Avenue. We were putting up Dean Roke's posters, and a bunch of white guys came out of a barroom and got in a real fight with us. The police arrested some of the guys that were in the fight but they left the white guys alone. They took the black ones down to Station Nine, and they beat up a couple of them. We ran up and told Dean about it. Dean at that time was a brilliant lawyer, and he had some pretty influential white people backing him financially. He picked up the phone and he got these people in on this thing, and the black guys were released right away. That was the first time I seen politics work . . . you know . . . pull . . . I couldn't believe it. I said, "Damn, look at this . . . a phone call to the right guy and wham." Them cops were bowing and scraping and apologizing.

So we started an Old Town Civic Club; part of it today is Freedom House. The other part is strictly political—Dean Roke clan. We started that thing. We sat down in Dean's office one night, and we talked about how if we could control some of those seats, the kinds of beautiful things that could happen to black people in Old Town.

So I said, "That's the road to go." I remembered all of the stuff from my childhood days, all the name-calling, the bigotry of the teachers, the sugar-coated way the school guidance counselors told you you couldn't do this or that because you were black. I got to saying to myself, "Gee, if we could get a foothold in politics, we could open the door to better education, we could kick some of these bigoted teachers out and put in some people that are really concerned."

It was at that time I went to live in the Garden Park Housing Project in East City, and I got a job there working with Housing as a janitor. I worked as a janitor for three years and then became a watchman. It was political pull that got me into Housing because at that time you couldn't get a job there without pull. I hurt my back on the job and was out of work for a year. When I was better, I started working in the boiler room as a fireman in the Bracken Field Housing Project. There was no transportation from where I lived, I had to be on the job early, I didn't have a car, so they moved me into Bracken Field. That's how I came to live here twelve years ago.

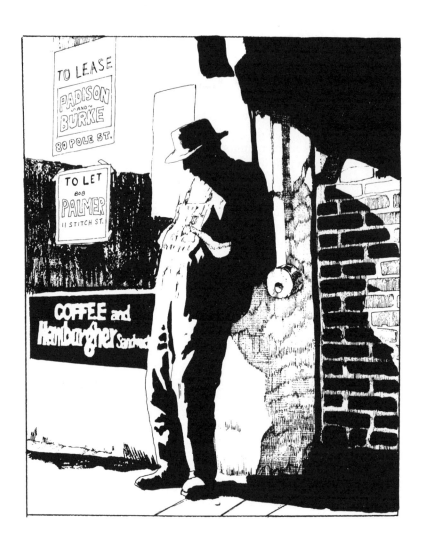

Mark Clay — Community Leader

*I had a deep affection and admiration for Mark Clay. He had
limited formal education but possessed an innate wisdom and understanding of people that was rare. He chaired many Community
Action Program meetings I attended, and I marvelled at his skill.*

*Mark grew up in the South, served in the Navy, went to prison
for six months for non-support of a child later proved not to be his,
had an unsuccessful marriage and a son before he came to live in
Bracken Field. He spoke to me at length about his life—never with
the least trace of bitterness. When I met him he was still working as
a laborer—I steered him to a job with one of the hospitals responsible for our program, and he became their first director of community relations. More than any other individual in Bracken Field,
Mark taught me how true participation in community affairs
enhances personality growth.*

I got really involved with community issues about ten years ago
when I moved into Bracken Field. I had started a program that I
was running myself, showing movies for the kids on Saturdays—
fifteen cents for four hours which was a pretty good baby-sitting
fee! And then I joined the United Voters League because I got interested in politics from the point of view of educating people how
to vote.

Then the Poverty Program came along, and that's when we really got involved because it was going to change the whole system
of government. They were going to bring in programs to help poor
people get out of their poverty cycle. I've always enjoyed a
challenge, so I tried to find out what it was all about. I wanted to
bring that program into the housing development so black people
could get involved. Black people were not getting involved when
the programs originally started in West Hill.

When the job of community organizer came up, I saw myself
as being more helpful working in the organization and I applied, but
I didn't get the job. Ned Handler got the job because he had a couple of years of college, and he had done some community work
with the National Association for the Advancement of Colored
People. But about a month later, I ended up the person who
became the boss. I didn't get the job of community organizer, but I
did get elected president which made me Ned's boss. I was unpaid
because none of the board members were paid. I was a factory

worker during the day and an office administrator at night. I was in
the board office eight hours every night making sure it ran right. I
was office manager, chairman of the board, contractor, carpenter,
I did everything. I spent as much time working for the CAP as I did
working at my regular job. I wanted it to work out because I felt
that this was the mechanism for poor people to do something, to
progress and get themselves out of poverty. I thought of this as the
answer to all of our problems. You know, everybody we hired were
community people, and they were doing a job and we had the
money to do that job. I thought, "Here's a chance for us to do
something the way we want to do it."

When I became the president of CAP, I recognized it as a
tremendous responsibility, and I began to really work at it. I used
to read all of the guidelines from headquarters over and over again
until I felt I had a fairly good understanding of what it meant. They
were telling us how we could spend the money, how we couldn't
spend the money, who could be on the board of directors, who
couldn't be on the board of directors, the income criteria, and the
different types of programs that we could get funded. I didn't know
nothing about parliamentary procedure, or I knew vaguely, but
most of the professionals on the board were very helpful in getting
me going. Like one of them wrote up a couple of sheets outlining
the duties of the chairman and how to run a meeting, about motions
and all that. At first nobody from Bracken Field knew how to write
proposals, and we relied very heavily on the professionals' opinions. We had a couple of professionals who were really on the
community's side, and they were very helpful to me with their advice.

My original thought of the Poverty Program was here was
money being allocated so that we could do things to better our community, and with this I could see playgrounds, tot lots, all different
kinds of athletic activities, and, frankly, the thing I had in mind was
a competitive type athletic program, city-wide, that would
particularly involve people and kids who live in housing projects.
But it wasn't the type of thing that the Office of Economic Opportunity was going with then. They were not funding recreation
type programs on a year-round basis, and they weren't giving
enough money for these programs to be self-sustaining. It's really
hard to get anything for kids out of OEO programs unless it's
something that they are running centrally, like the Neighborhood
Youth Corps, or the Job Corps or something which is really job
oriented.

The ones that are my biggest concern are the teenagers because everybody's against teenagers. Everybody talks about teenagers doing this and that and when they open their mouths and want to speak, nobody listens—"Well what do you know about it, you're only a kid." I've always been for the underdog, or the kid on the block whom nobody likes because he's dirty or he's ragged, or he's poor, or he has a speech impediment, or he walks with a limp—this is the kid I've always had a lot of time for. In that age group, from fifteen years and up, there are so many lonely people. If you can get a place open, like a teen center or a teen lounge, . . . everybody says you've got to have some kind of constructive program . . . I say they just want to go there to hang out . . .

I guess when you're chairman, you get to see some things happen, for instance, when you go down to the central office you meet people from other areas and talk about what's going on in their area, and people call you with new ideas, and the type of guy I am I never give myself a moment's rest. Even when I was sitting watching TV, I'd be thinking about what I could do to make the organization better, or what kind of program could we really get going, and was it feasible to do this or that. I'd try to figure out the best ways to go about any new idea I got, like who to contact in order to get things moving; so I guess you might say I became a strategist and tried to develop strategy in fulfilling a goal.

For me it was a real education. I learned to understand myself better. I really got confidence in myself that I could do something other than manual labor because I ran meetings, and because I had been to meetings and because of the way the program at CAP was going. I found out that I had fairly good common sense and was able to make rational decisions, and one of the biggest things I found out about myself was that I enjoy helping people, I enjoy being an advocate for people. If somebody's got a problem or a fight, I enjoy picking up the fight and going with them. It was a tremendous education just to deal with the East City Central Antipoverty Office. They would tell our staff, "you don't represent the community . . . we don't have to talk to you. You get the CAP Board down here." They'd tell our Board, "you don't understand, you've got all that staff out there, why isn't your staff doing thus and so," and they'd play one against the other. So when they'd write memos, we'd write memos too.

The Poverty Program, the OEO program, has produced a lot of people that were hiding under the rug, so to speak, that had talent to do things, and it really brought them out. An enormous number of black people would probably still be in a factory some place, or in a ditch, or in somebody's kitchen, taking care of somebody's children out in the suburbs someplace if this Community Action or OEO program hadn't come along. I don't know where I would be if this hadn't happened to come along, and even though I had this confidence in myself to run the West Hill CAP, it took much longer for me to get confidence in myself that I could do a job and be *paid* to do something else. This is one of the biggest things that the Poverty Program has produced. A lot of people like me who got enough confidence in themselves to say, "I'm going to get out of this factory and stop being underemployed." It has brought a lot of people who were underemployed up to their full potential.

In Bracken Field I feel like I'm the Joneses, and I think that every community should have its Joneses, because if you don't have Joneses then everybody gets in the same rut, or gets in real apathy, and don't try to do any better, don't try to progress. So, as long as I can project something to other people, I feel like I'm really doing something. In the housing project some of the older teenagers and people in general remember that I was working in a factory, and I had a really tough job, and they can see that there's somebody that's picked himself up by the bootstraps, and I have the respect of the people in the community. Like people stop me on the street and tell me their boy is so and so and getting in trouble, and they can't handle him, and would I speak to him, and kids tell me their fathers can't handle them, and would I have a talk with their fathers. It's for these reasons that I won't move out of the housing project as long as they'll let me stay, no matter how much money I'm making.

Mabel Straley — A Pillar of Strength

Mabel Straley is a person to whom others go for help in times of stress. She is a natural leader, a willing worker, a fighter for others' rights. Mabel is on just about every organization in Bracken Field. A busy, happy wife and mother, she has enough energy left over to take on the cares of the housing project, particularly those of its beleaguered youth.

I see myself as a facilitator in groups because there are lots of community people who've never had exposure to groups. If they see people who appear to know everything they think, "I'm not going to say anything because it will look foolish coming from me." If I lead off with a suggestion, then automatically everybody's going to say, "Oh, that's a good idea," and follow it, but if I keep prodding them, they'll join in the talk about problems themselves.

Sometimes it's difficult for me because people see me as the Community Action Program. I don't know whether it's a power struggle or whether it's because people feel inadequate themselves, but they have this definite feeling about CAP. I'm the CAP Center Coordinator, and responsible for staff activities in this area. I live in the area, and I've been with CAP almost from the time it started in 1964.

Before I joined CAP, I was a member of the United Voters League which was formed to give political education to the community. Robert Prescott headed it. It was the only viable community organization in the area at that time. I joined the United Voters League because I wanted to know more about politics relevant to the community . . . I was looking for something that would make the community a better place to live in. When the poverty program was introduced, members of the United Voters League and some others acted as an ad hoc committee to bring the poverty program into the area. I was on that ad hoc committee as was Robert Prescott, and Mark Clay and others.

I took a job with CAP as a community worker because I'd always been involved and interested in community affairs, and I was already doing this kind of work, but it was very difficult to get out of the house—to tell my husband I had this meeting or that meeting to attend. Also I had a baby, and instead of dragging him to meetings with me, I could pay someone to take care of him. I would be able to do all kinds of things I really liked to do and add some.

When CAP first opened its doors we did a survey of the entire community needs and listed what people voiced as a desire to have in the community. The number one priority was a library—a study hall for the youth. Mark Clay built the bookshelves, the youth and men came together to stain them and do the floors—it was a real community project. CAP pays the salaries of three library aides and a supervisor to run the library. Another program we started was the tutoring program—it's worked out beautifully—we're always swamped with applications. Of course we didn't get everything people wanted. For instance, people wanted a day care center large enough to accomodate all the children whose mothers wanted to go to work. And they wanted better police protection. They asked for better recreational facilities, and for a while it seemed that Housing and the Park Department were going to put in a beautiful recreational center, but it never materialized.

We managed to get enough signatures of residents to get the university's well baby clinic moved from the neighborhood hall to its present location. The community was very proud when those doors first opened, and they had this nice clean baby clinic . . . it was really something.

CAP has done a lot. OEO looks for statistics, but what I look at is what would be left if CAP pulled out today? The most important thing that comes to mind is the kind of leaders that CAP has helped to develop. If there is any kind of problem in our community today, there are people who know how to deal with it. CAP has introduced them to agencies . . . helped them to develop skills . . . the kind of things that money won't buy. I think in terms of leaders like Robert Prescott and Mark Clay among others. Robert Prescott who has made valuable contributions to education concepts . . . community involvement in education. Mark Clay who just wanted to take the weight of the whole community on his shoulders and really did. Others like our receptionist who became a Headstart teacher. These people were looking for something to use up their energy.

Getting people out to attend meetings—that's the most difficult job of all. You can't blame them. At home they have so many problems. Unless you can solve their immediate problems, they don't want to come. But as each new group is formed, even if we get just two new people, it's a step forward. Even if we only reach people through flyers, they gain some knowledge. Eventually a lot of people are reached and can begin to do things on their own. Many people have gone through training programs . . . they became motivated . . . they moved out of the area . . . they purchased their own homes . . . they changed their jobs. It's not things you can write down . . . it's not statistics that the government may have . . . but it's there.

I was eighteen when I got married, and I had five children. My husband had been married before, and I looked after his two children also. Four of my children were "premies," but pregnancy was always a happy time for me. My oldest daughter is going to college next year, but she hasn't yet decided what she wants to be. The fourteen year old is more aggressive . . . she'll do well I think. They all do very well at school but my fourteen year old says, "Mommy, I'm a low achiever because there's nothing that really fits my needs." I'm in the process of finding a community school that might be more challenging for her. I try to build up self-confidence in my children so that they can determine what's right for them, and then map out a pattern of how they can reach it. It's a hard job because I live in the housing project but so far it's worked out pretty well. We've been pretty lucky.

My oldest stepson became an addict three years ago. I was glad that he had enough strength, enough love, to come to me and ask for help. He went to the hospital. They say they cure them. But once they're addicts, they have to fight to survive every day of their lives, and it's really a sad thing. Parents know their kids have problems, but they don't want to admit it because they don't know what to do about it. My stepson's still fighting it.

I guess I was always aware of peoples' problems. I always had that determination that I was going to do something about things that affected me. The first thing I really did like that was during the Korean conflict when I wrote to President Eisenhower protesting the treatment of some of the guys in the Infantry that were mobilized from my area. After that I was president of the National Baptist Youth Fellowship Group. And then I moved into the housing development and into work with the United Voters League and the War on Poverty Program. I had lots of exposure to community problems, and I guess I was always a leader. I felt that we were as equal as anybody else and we should fight for anything that affected us.

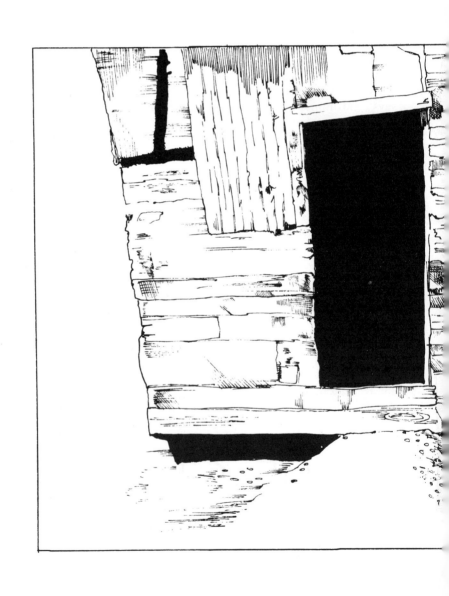

Chapter IV

Project Youth

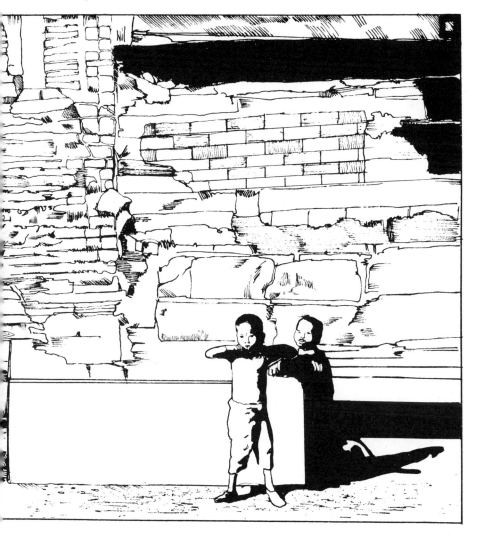

Sandra Richards — Identity Seeker

*Sandra worked for me as an interviewer our first summer at the
Health Center, helping collect census data in Bracken Field. I kept
her on, thereafter, as my research assistant while she struggled
with doubts about the worth of continuing her college education.*

*Since childhood Sandra had wanted to be a doctor. I could
have helped her choose and be admitted to a good medical school,
had she not decided against completing the necessary premedical
requirements. For two years Sandra seesawed between the intellectualism of the white university world and the solidarity of a
black separatist group before she finally left us. I loved her, but I
never fully reached her.*

It was the beginning of spring . . . around March when I came to
your office, and I decided to come to Bracken Field Health Center.
That summer I worked for you, I got involved in your census survey, and I guess it was a complete turning around in my life. Since
then I've been involved in a lot of health organizations, and I've
met a lot of people.

For instance, I was invited to attend meetings a community
group from my area had started to discuss the suggested group
health plan the university wanted to introduce. At the beginning,
the main function of that committee was to decide on the site of a
community outreach (satellite) health unit for the university. This
was to placate the community which was up in arms about the fact
that the clinic proposed for them had been part of the downtown
clinic rather than a separate clinic in their own neighborhood.

I got elected secretary at that first meeting. From then on, I
went to all the big meetings and took notes and tried to soothe tem-
pers and tried to change the outlook of the people. At the beginning, they were really provincial and parochial—they could only
think of themselves as helpmates to the university, and I and a few
of the people argued, I think successfully, that their commitment
was to the community, not to the university, and that they should
look beyond the university to other sources of medical care for the
community; that the university at most would only enroll a certain
percentage of the community.

The committee has really grown in their outlook—they're now
five times more militant and more together than they were when I
first came to the meetings. Not too long ago, they had a confrontation with the director of the plan to demand independence for the

committee. They wanted their own budget so that they could do things on their own. As it is now, we have to send out our letters through the university—they pay all the postage and everything, and whenever we want any petty cash, we have to make a formal request and negotiate for only ten dollars.

The university's plans for the outreach center didn't really coincide with the committee's feelings. The committee wanted a doctor . . . they wanted a mini-comprehensive health center . . . a community outreach center. The doctors did not want to have a physician in the outreach center—they wanted to put a social worker there and perhaps a nurse, and bus people downtown for medical care. But now there will be some physician services in the outreach center which shows you the power of the community— it's a complete turn-around from the position that the physicians had.

There were some things I didn't like when I worked with the committee. A lot of the committee members were so mercenary that it was really shameful. Delia Holder got mad because she felt they were after her job. A lot of the committee people want to be hired as community workers by the university. They want to be co-opted by the Establishment. I just don't understand it.

It's sort of unfair, too, because there are other people in the community who might be even more suited or who might work harder. It's pretty bad for people to get on a committee solely to get a job. For months, this attitude has been showing. In the middle of a meeting, someone will start asking about benefits when we've been talking on a subject that has nothing at all to do with that. It's out of place, and I think it's morally wrong. If you're on a committee, doing something for the community should be the foremost thing on your mind, and employment or money should be secondary. But the committee is growing a lot more sophisticated now.

My own background? I was born in Montogomery, Alabama, but I didn't live there very long. My father was in the Navy, and we moved several times before we came to East City. I'm the oldest of ten kids.

I lived with my grandmother in Buffalo, off and on for three or four years at a time. She accepted me like her daughter and was very overprotective. I felt that the only way I could achieve independence and learn to be an adult would be to leave Buffalo, so I came back to East City.

My mother was born in the South in a fairly well-to-do family. They had a lot of land and everything in Montgomery. My father's family was a lot poorer. He comes from the South, too, from a small town . . . people have chickens and things like that, a train goes through, and there's coal fields nearby.

I guess I had a different upbringing with my grandmother because I'm a lot different from my sisters and brothers and from most of the people I know. Like I have respect for older people— they have none at all.

My mother went to college and got a Bachelor's degree, but she took a job as a secretary in a newspaper office—that's all. My father finished high school and then went into the Navy where he stayed for twenty years. We had a pretty good life; we could afford anything we wanted; we had a father and a mother; we were never on welfare; we always had books, had to do our homework, and follow rules and regulations.

There were problems in my relationship with my mother. There's always been a feud between my mother and my grandmother. It was already there before I was born, but my grandmother was crazy about me and my mother felt that the only way she could get back at her was to strike through me. That was one of the reasons why I went to Buffalo a lot. Now that I'm grown, it's in the past and forgiven, but I can't really forget.

My mother leans on me now to take care of all the other kids, but when I was younger, I got the feeling that I must be doing something wrong. I kept trying to figure out why she should be punishing me if I hadn't done anything. I tried to overcompensate for guilt feelings by trying to be better than all the other kids . . . to work harder than all of them. It was pretty difficult.

At high school I belonged to the clique . . . the smartest kids . . . the ones who took all the honors subjects. We were members of the Honors Society; we put on the school shows; we were on the debating team. I joined practically all the clubs and was an officer in all of them. I wasn't with the other kids that much socially because I couldn't get out, so I made up for it in school and after school activities. I didn't even date till I was seventeen or so. For the most part, I was around adults.

In the South, the way to advance was to become a school teacher. Nobody in our family ever thought of becoming a doctor. But from when I was a little kid, I never thought about being a social worker, or a teacher, or anything else but a doctor. Now I'm not so sure. The roles in today's world are changing so rapidly, it's very hard to decide just what you want to be. Also I found out I like other things.

I used to want to be a noble person in life . . . you know, saving everybody. I got pretty disillusioned when I started reading medical journals and saw all those horrible advertisements in there, and the crass materialism. Until recently, I've had a sort of onesided view of the doctor . . . sort of a mystical person. I guess the reason why I really got interested in it was because I was fascinated by life and death, and I wanted to learn more about it. Ever since I was young, I was fascinated by the forces that shape us, life and death, what pain is, and things like that.

I was a bright kid, but they never really thought anybody in our family would go to college. My mother had gone, but that was down South, and her parents had had money to send her. There was never any poor people going to college.

By the time I got out of high school, I wasn't really that enthusiastic about going to college, but I came to East City, and once there I decided that, "Well, what the heck." I had an interview at North University and forgot all about it until I got a letter that said that I won a scholarship. I said, "How can this be? . . . I hadn't even applied for it, so how could I win one?" Then I decided, "I'll go to college."

I didn't feel it was really a university . . . really we were getting paid to integrate the college. It was like a factory, turning out people and sending them off to industry. It was horrible. All we did was to cram, and there was never time to learn anything or to read for any of the subjects.

We were on a work-study program—all the kids were given jobs to help them out financially. That's when I worked in a social science research organization. I got a really bad impression of research because it was so badly done. They turned out all sorts of junk—you wondered why they were doing research. The organization did a lot of sex research. It was a strange place. Anyhow, I learned about key-punching, and I went to a course on programming. After that I found my own jobs. The university was supposed to match the jobs to the students' interests, but the difference between rhetoric and practice was long. For example, English majors got jobs in clinics!

The only course I really enjoyed was a history course I took with a professor who was really nice. I wrote a paper for him on the theme of Negro discrimination from 1930-1950, and at the end of the report, I put down some of my experiences as a child. Doing that brought it all back to me, and I found it very hard to go back to classes and to be around those people.

I remembered incidents when I travelled with my grandmother, sitting in a special section of the train—which was dirty—and not being able to buy food in restaurants when we were hungry. I remembered all the times since then when I'd gone into a store to buy something, getting my change on the counter while white people got it given in their hand. You get discriminated against so much you forget about it—it's part of daily living—until something happens that really angers you, and then you remember the thousand other times this happened. The fact that you can't get a cab, you accept, but when you actually get into a cab, and the driver refuses to take you where you're going, you get mad.

I'm very good friends with a fellow who's head of the Black Student Association, and I get along well with what people call the radical, militant part of the black population, although I'm out of touch with them presently. A year ago, I was really bitter, and I wanted to go to Nigeria. It seemed horrible just to be in this country, and I wondered what it would be like to go to a country where the majority of the people are black. I was bitter because of things I read in Black Panther newspapers and because a lot of my friends had been beaten up. Then I would forget again until something happened to bring it all back.

People don't have any idea of the depth of hate and bitterness that young kids have . . . it's really fantastic. Many young black kids are very, very militant . . . very, very anti-white. I feel schizoid because I have a lot of white friends.

I'm thinking of going to Jamaica. I'm in a quandary. Young college kids are the ones who are really confused about what to do. Should we go to school, or go into industry and get jobs and just do the same old thing? Should we become revolutionary, put on khakis and work for the community? Or what do we do? Young people who are radically different are a minority . . . the majority of kids are just like their ma and pa. They go into business, go to school, study hard, while the other kids are picketing. Really concerned people are out in the street while everybody else goes to classes.

I'm not sure what I'm going to do. I'm not sure if I'm going back to college or not. I'll probably become a mad programmer. But I'll continue to work with community groups—probably more intensively.

Claude — A Future Lawyer

Claude resembles one of the young black teenagers described by Sandra who bears a deep resentment to the white world. He is unusual in Bracken Field since from the age of fourteen he has spent most of his spare time as a volunteer, working in the project's Community Center, where he has earned the respect and admiration of community leaders. He allowed me to interview him because Mark Clay interceded on my behalf, but he was uncomfortable, difficult to interview and guarded in his attitude towards me.

I used to live in Old Town, and I came to live in Bracken Field about four and a half years ago. There are eight of us in the family counting my parents. Three a piece, boys and girls. I'm third. My father is a printer. My mother doesn't work. We're not all that close a family.

I'm a senior in high school now. School is all right in the early years, but then the later you go, it tends to get boring, and you know, as you wake up to what's going on in school, you see the whole picture. There are a lot of sides to the school that you don't know about. There are some prejudiced teachers, but if I go and tell my parents that, well, this teacher flunked me because I'm black, they will say, "Well, you just didn't do your homework," or "Your must have been acting up." They don't tend to believe what the children say.

I don't know what I'm going to do when I finish school. I was planning to go to college, but as of right now, I don't know. If I do go to college, I'll probably study law because I feel like there are not enough black lawyers. And there's enough black people's problems so that we need strong representation in court. I know that from my own experience.

I got picked up five months ago for possession of marijuana. It happened like this. Myself and my friend, we met two white girls which we didn't know. I believe they had been drinking. I don't know for sure. They had a car, and they wanted to ride in the town. We were going in town, so we told them we'd show them how to get to the places they wanted to go. While we were going to town, the girls pulled out a bag of marijuana. The police stopped the car because he said we were driving in an unusual manner without the back lights on. When he stopped us, the girls put the marijuana under the front seat. The police made us get out of the car and he searched the car and found the marijuana. He charged me with possession and my friend with being present. He turned the two girls loose even though it was their car. The girls said they found the marijuana between my legs. And when my friend got to court, he was also charged with possession. When the judge asked the police what happened to the two girls, he said he turned them loose because he believed what they said. I got six months probation, and my friend was fined fifty dollars. So that's an example of what I mean right there.

In a sense the project is like a jail. Everything that goes on in the project tends to spread inside the project, but not much outside the project. If you were to try and get away from me (if you lived in the project), your will power wouldn't be that strong for you to be able to do that. Even if you left the project to get away from the crowd there, sooner or later you'd be coming back because your friends are there.

I'm different, not because I've only been in the project four years, you know, it's the same all over. . .maybe it's just the way I am. I had my share of seeing the street life. 'Cause like, they do say you learn more off the street than you do in school. And there's a lot of things on the street which people don't realize you know about. You might learn about stealing cars, and then again you might learn about what the consequences are of stealing cars because you seen what happened to this man over here. If you want to get to the teenagers, you can't do it by just having a new building and an organization over here and expect the teenagers to come into it. They're out in the street doing their little thing, so you have to get to them through the street. Parents tend to say, "My son wouldn't do this. . .my daughter wouldn't do this," so you can't really talk to parents unless they change their whole attitude.

I'm trying to look after my younger brother and my sisters. I talk to them just like I talk to anybody else where I work at the Community Center. I started working at the Community Center after the community took it over, and I've been there about a year and a half now. I work there full time in the summer and after school part-time during the school year. There are a lot of temptations in the project. It's easier to fall into the bad things than into the good. There's not much recreational facilities, but there's a gym in the Community Center which has been getting a lot of kids off the street, plus the Cellar. The Cellar is like a teen center—our school kids are down there half the time. The Cellar is mainly recreational now, but it's gonna grow to the point where it's gonna be educational, too.

I'm not really sure what I'll be doing next year, as I said before, but I know I'll stay in the type of work that means I'll be working with people. If I become a lawyer, I won't work with the big individual. I mean I won't work with the man with the money, the man who goes in and gets ahead and tries to stay ahead 'cause he's got some money. Those men tend to get behind a desk and forget about things they went through. They forget their parents and the things other people are going through now.

Is living in the housing project better or worse than living in Old Town? Well, I don't know. When you first move some place different things are strange and you don't know many people. In a sense it's better than Old Town 'cause like in the project everybody's living tight, close together in a small area. That way you know many more people, and you have more fun knowing more people. Moving from the project wouldn't be all that much better. The houses would be further apart, and you wouldn't get that same feeling you get in the project having somebody next door that you may be close with. The project is like one big family. I like to live where there are lots of people.

I play basketball and I also like to read. I read black books— books by black authors about black people. The last one I read was *Native Son,* by Richard Wright. I started Cleaver's *Soul on Ice,* I started *Malcolm X,* but I never did get around to finishing them. I read some white authors who write mystery or suspense, but I really like to read black authors. It's just where I am. I'm black myself, and I believe black people can get across a point to me better than a white person. Yuh, I'm proud of being black, and I want to bring it out more.

One thing I'd like to do for the teenagers of Bracken Field is teach them black awareness. And that knowledge is power, so they ought to stay in school. I would take time to let them know that they have to do things for themselves first, before they can expect to get out and do things for somebody else. They've got to get themselves some place first, before they can help the next person. If even one person in the project really got some place, in the sense of owning his own business, he could turn back, if he was that type of person, and offer the rest jobs that they would be able to fit in.

Tom — A Pragmatic Maintenance Worker

Tom was introduced to me as a youth I might be interested in interviewing—he had been one of the "bad guys" and was now reformed. I had not met him before and was surprised at his candor. Tom did not have unrealistic expectations of himself. He was concerned about the needs of his younger siblings and indeed of all the adolescents who lived in the housing project. He impressed me as a youth who, maturing late, would probably stay out of trouble and with luck would achieve some of his future ambitions.

When I moved to East City, I started getting into trouble; I've been here seven or eight years now. I was twelve when I came here, and I met a lot of guys and started getting into trouble with them. One night I stole a car.

I got caught. I went to court. They put me on probation, and I stayed out of trouble for two or three years. Then I started hanging out in the project again. I didn't have no job, or nothing, just hung around in the streets, like everybody else, and I got in trouble again. Used to go around snatching pocketbooks, beating up people, stealing their money and all kinds of things like that. I had a fight with somebody . . . they called it assault and battery . . . went to court . . . they put me on Youth Service Board. After that I stopped getting into trouble for a couple of years, and then I got a job in the project. As soon as I got that job with East City Housing, as maintenance worker in the project, I haven't been in no more trouble.

I used to buy reefer with the money I stole, marijuana. I started smoking it before I was sixteen, and then I started smoking hash. Some of them guys buy smack, and usually they shoot it up in their veins. I never tried it. I smoked marijuana, but I never touched heroin, because I seen a guy one day, I seen him pass out 'cause he took too much of it. I might have tried it, but I would never touch it after I seen that.

Everybody else was smoking pot, and it seemed like it wasn't nothing else they was doing . . . wasn't nothing else to do. Just sit around and play cards all day; there was no basketball court or nothing like that, the playground is all messed up.

I think everybody in the United States smokes pot. It's like smoking a cigarette, it's not habit forming or nothing. And it's just another way of taking a drink of beer, or whiskey, or champagne.

It's the same thing. I don't see nothing wrong with it. I even think the President does it. It's better than drinking because drinking does something to your insides and marijuana doesn't. I think you have a better chance on marijuana than you do on liquor.

Well, I used to smoke it all day, you know . . . cut it. I had nothing to do, I was kind of shy. Smoke a little bit of it and I'd feel kind of happy, didn't worry about nothing. And it made us think a little harder. Like if somebody said, "Let's go do something," we'd start thinking, "Will I get in trouble if I do this?", so then maybe you don't do it. You just have a little smoke and start some music and sit outside and listen to the music until you get tired and go home and to to sleep. There's nothing wrong with it. Yeah, you have to steal to buy it, but I usually never bought none . . . one of the guys bought it and I got it from him.

The kids that go around now snatching pocketbooks do it for the money, because they got hooked on that smack and now they have a Jones [withdrawal symptoms] behind it. They have to keep up their habit, but they don't have no money so they have to go out and make it somewhere. Like I've got a friend, just got out of jail two days ago. He snatched a pocketbook four years ago and stayed in jail for four years. He came out a couple of days ago, and he's snatching pocketbooks again. Nowadays the guys that go around robbing and stealing steal because if they don't keep up their habit, they might get sick. They don't want the Jones to come on. They have either to kick the habit or just keep on going, and most of them are scared of kicking.

Kids start at ten, eleven on up. Kids of all ages take everything. Some of them sniff it, the first time, then they find out it messes up the brain or something, and they stop that. Then maybe they start shooting it, and after that they're hooked. The average kid today that shoots up smack is around fourteen years old.

Most of the kids there now, they're trying to kick the habit. A couple of kids have kicked it already. There's only about a dozen or so now on dope in the project. Something has helped; it may be the Health Center, 'cause once they seen this boy, Wally, he went into the hospital first, and then he kicked the habit, so they all started going to the drug unit in the health center. Once the kids see the big kids are stopping, they aren't going to try it.

The kids need some kind of activities around here. Some of the kids have nothing to do, no place to go. We used to have the Cellar for the older kids—I used to work down there. We tried to get some educational programs going but the kids just wanted to shoot pool, play records and dance. It got closed down, and after a month everybody forgot about the place and didn't want to go back. When it opened again later, they gave it to the little kids, the youngsters. There's supposed to be a meeting this afternoon to try and plan some bus trips for the older kids, you know, at night time. I'm supposed to go over to help arrange them. And that might help some. I think if they got a lot of new programs going that the teenagers would be interested in they wouldn't have so much problems.

You want to know about school? I finished the tenth grade, and I was going to the eleventh when I got that job in the project with East City Housing; that's what changed my mind. I liked school, it was pretty good, but when I got the job making that kind of money, I figured if I finish high school I'll probably only make the same amount, so I stayed on the job. But I don't like the way the school system's set up around here. The teachers are prejudiced and everything, and the school system is all messed up. When I was going to school I used to get suspended every week. I might forget my tie or something, or get into trouble with a girl, or have a fight in school, something like that. The teachers kept bugging you and bugging you, and they come out with that stick, that rattan, and they beat you to death with that. And when your parents come, they cook up a whole lot of lies.

When I first started going to high school, it was a good school. Then they got these young kids that just come out of college, you know, these hippie teachers and what not, they don't know what's going on. When they start teaching for the first year, they don't know what they're doing. They think they might say the wrong thing, and it might upset somebody, and then cause a big feud. For instance, they've got two guys fighting in the corner. The young teacher is scared. If he goes over there and touches them, he might get punched in the mouth or something. He's supposed to try and break it up whether he gets hurt or not; he's supposed to try and do his job. You need rough teachers that really know how to get down on the kids to make them stop fighting, instead of just beating them on the hands. That ain't going to do anything but just make them worse.

Books? No. I never liked to read. I never read no books. I read the funnies in the paper. Or the horoscope part. The only time I read the news is if something happens overnight, like somebody getting shot or something like that. I watch TV when the basketball season starts . . . I watch the games. I watch every game on TV. And I watch the Rock and Roll shows. And I watch some games they have in the morning like Concentration, and Jeopardy and things like that. I don't like to watch no love stories or nothing like that.

The people the kids look up to? There's a guy who's supposed to be the baddest guy in the project, and all the kids look out and say, "Well, I want to be like him when I get big. I want to be mean like him, I want to go shoot dope like him every day." They probably like the way he's dressed, you know, the way he talks and the way he goes around and bullies people to get what he wants without going through a lot of hassle. He just says, "Give it to me," and they give it to him. And they say, "Well, that's the easy way to do it." So they want to do it like that. But if he stops doing it, gets hurt or something, they're going to want to stop also.

The majority follow the bad guys. They push dope, they take dope, sell all kinds of dope. The community doesn't stop them because they're scared. They're scared if they do something, they might get some of their friends and hurt them. I used to be that way when I was a kid. I wanted to be a bad guy too. I wanted to do anything I didn't have to work for. I just wanted to sit back and collect money and never work.

You want money because you see a big car . . . you want a brand new car. You think, "Well I could get this and that." Then when I got that job over here two years ago, it changed my whole mind about everything 'cause I get money every week now, and I don't have to go out and steal no money now. And if I need a car, I can go out and rent a car. If I want to buy something, I can go buy it. See, once you get a job, making money, you don't need to go out and steal nothing. If every guy in the project there had a job, I think at least one hundred and fifty dollars a week, there wouldn't be no problems.

I have six brothers and sisters, and I'm not worried about them. I keep my younger brother away from the bad guys. I know who to let him hang out with and who not to. I think a boy needs a man in the house, a father or somebody that's really going to get down on him. My father's been living with me all his life, and he still lives with me. He doesn't work now. He had an accident, and

he's disabled. I get along with him. But he clamped down on me real hard. He seemed to me kind of mean, you know, when I was
young. That's life. Everybody needs real parents. Who wants to be
living with someone who's going to stay for one year, and then the
next year somebody else moves in? The kids don't go along with
that. When that starts happening, then they start hating their
mother. They don't know what to do. They might want to kill that
guy, or the mother or something like that. It drives the kids crazy.

When I have kids, I don't want to be living here. I'd like them
to have a nice house out in the country somewhere where there's
not too many kids. A house with a lot of grass so they can have a
place to play. A next door neighbor maybe, but not too many people, just, quiet. Then you can raise your kids up right, 'cause
there's nobody there but you and your next door neighbor. So
that's what I hope, that's what I want. It's hard for kids to grow up
in the city. I'd like my kids to go to school, finish school, and go to
college. Because these guys that are getting out of high school,
they make the same amount I make, but the guys getting out of college they're making good money. They got a lot going for them. So
I'd rather my kids go all the way.

If I could get money, I'd put more money into the community.
Like the project—it's dirty. I'd get more guys at work in there; I'd
put more in so they'd get paid. And have the place cleaned up, have
it looking nice like it used to look eight years ago. It's the people,
the tenants. They don't care. They send their little kids out to the
incinerator, little kids this small with big bags, they can't open the
thing and put the bag in. They just leave it by the incinerator. Then
a dog comes along and rips the bag open. There's garbage all over
the place. People are too lazy to come down with their garbage,
they throw it out of the windows. They don't have enough dis-
cipline.

And another thing. Mr. Prescott from the manager's office
sent a letter to every parent in the project, and said that if anybody
gets caught buying hot goods from these guys they're going to be
evicted from the project. I go along with that one hundred percent.
If they wouldn't buy the stuff the guys stoled, they couldn't do
nothing with it but just keep it, and it's not going to do them no
good just keeping it.

Organizations? There's too many organizations in Bracken
Field. The Health Center's all right. Everybody over here uses the

Health Center. When I get sick or something that's the first place I go to. I don't want to spend no carfare to go way down to East City Hospital. But the other organizations—all they do is fight. Like if one's getting some money and another organization finds out about it, they want to get the money also, and they're fighting each other. I saw this happen. But I guess we should have more black people in politics. I think there's a lot of black people that's eligible for it, but they just don't get the jobs.

Chapter V

Health Center Community Workers

Mrs. King — A Community Health Worker

Dignified but smiling, tall, plump and big bosomed, Mrs. King personified warmth, comfort and motherliness. Despite the hardships of her life and a growing sophistication, Mrs. King never lost the gentleness of her rural Sourthern upbringing. Too proud to ask for help for herself, she instinctively responded to the needs of others. Her warm personality admirably suited her job as community health worker.

I was born in North Carolina in a small town. It's a pretty little town, and to me my childhood was one of the happiest childhoods that anybody ever had. We were a very close family. I used to enjoy waking up in the morning . . . you could hear the birds singing . . . I've never seen a morning in East City like it. We had a dog and a duck, and we had a nice lawn with big trees where we played.

My father is a Minister and my life was surrounded by church. I had one brother and two sisters, four of us, and all my family and my father's family and my mother's family are close together. My mother loved people, so we always had someone staying with us. There was a lot of girls went to school there, from the country, and my mother would let them come to her house to go to school. North Carolina is a state that really pushed education, but we didn't get it.

I think the South is a much better place than a lot of people say it is. I know there's a lot of things wrong there, but if the whites don't like it, they'll let you know. They don't hold it in. We knew we couldn't go into the drugstore to have a coke. When I came to East City, if you went into a place, they let you go in but you sat an hour before they served you. Of course North Carolina was a place for cotton. I hated picking cotton. But today they have machines to do the work. There's a more relaxed living. I don't think everybody's so rushed, but I can't compare it from when I lived there till now because it has changed.

My mother insisted that we finish high school, and I finished high school. I wanted to go to nurse's school, but I didn't have a good school system at home—most of the teachers were people that you knew and they automatically passed you; so I didn't get that good a schooling. My C average wasn't good enough, and they

wouldn't accept me at Wilmington; so I went to Baltimore. I went
to the University Hospital there as a nurse aide.

I met my husband while I was working in Virginia during the
war. He was a sailor. His home was in Massachusettes, near
Falmouth. He said he wouldn't like to live in the South, but he was
in Charleston when he was in the service.

I'm a little ashamed of where I live now, living in the project;
I'm ashamed for my family to come see where I'm living, and I
shouldn't be. Hallways not clean and elevators not clean. You
clean them out . . . we cleaned up last Saturday, and it's filthy
now, but after you get in and close the door, you can really enjoy
your apartment.

Sister Pat and Sister Mary live right across the street from me.
They have a car, and we all go shopping together. They came to my
son's party, and they are going to come sewing with us. Sister
Mary got robbed, you know, and now she is very afraid. When we
go out, we make sure we walk them up. It hurts to know that staying here anybody can get hurt . . . that's the sad thing about it. I
think the most saddest thing about anything around here is to see
the children that we know doing these bad things. We're going to
have to speak up and tell them that we know who they are. But I'm
afraid my children will get hurt if I do. Sometimes these bad boys
don't bother you, but they'll bother the children.

A lady I know said she did tell the police about one of the boys
who robbed, and the police said we have to *see* the boy doing it;
you can't convict a boy by hearsay. You could hurt a person if you
did because with the boys wearing Afros, they all look alike,
especially from the back. I know I've mistaken my own son for
another boy I thought was him, same height and everything.

They're stealing because they have to have enough money to
live. You know, now you're afraid to buy anything for the house,
because you don't know when you come back if it will be gone.
They're breaking into the homes too—it's like a barricade.

Mr. Prescott, the acting manager, had a building meeting. He
said something that was really important. He said we've got to stop
barricading ourselves and try to do something about vandalism.
We've got to listen for each other's door, instead of when we hear a
noise not answering and not saying a thing about it. I was really upset about having a building meeting. You don't know your own
neighbors . . . you don't know whether to let them in. Next day

they might come back and break in. But he said to try and get friendly with the neighbors. I live in a building with twenty-eight families, and it's more cold and not as friendly as a three-story building, because sometimes you only know the people on your own floor. But I think the best thing you can do is just to respect each other, though that's kind of hard to do when you live next door to children that has babies when they're not married.

I don't like being full of fear as I am now. Drugs is one of the things I'm afraid of. And fear I'm not giving my children a good start in life because of the environment here. Maybe you have to go back again with me to when I was a little girl. I guess it's the way I was raised. If you would drink and different things, well you stayed at that side, but if you wanted to be respected, you'd behave differently and be in another class. And that's the comparison I had with the project where everybody's mixed up together, and you can't tell who's who. And I'm afraid my children are going to be caught up in this same thing, if they're not strong enough to keep out of this. And you don't know who's moved in—that's what bothers me the most.

I'm afraid right next door to you people is selling drugs or using drugs, and the same children that was living there when I first moved in are the ones that's giving us the worst time here. They are the ones robbing the people and the ones that are taking the dope. And see, all these kids grew up together, and these kids will stick together. . .they know each other. My own might start taking the drugs. So far I haven't had the problem, but I don't know when it will start. Also, we're living with parents there that's selling these drugs to children. I guess I still have a fondness for the way I grew up, and maybe it's not right to try to push my children in that same pattern, but I just can't change. I feel that certain standards are certain standards, and I think you're judged by the company you keep.

Another thing. . .we didn't have to barricade our doors with locks and bolts when we first moved in. I used to take my daughter to kindergarten and leave my door open. And yet, and still, it's a nice place because you can make your apartment look so beautiful, and we don't get the opportunity as black people to get good houses. Where can you buy a house? The house you can buy is not really in good condition, and you're struggling the rest of your life trying to pay for it. But the project seems to be holding us down. When your children grow up and start working, the rent goes up, and you don't get a chance to save. You're always standing still—they add the children's salary onto what you make, and that makes the rent higher, and you're still the same.

I'm in a different predicament too. My husband worked for twelve years and now he's disabled. That's another reason we're still here. I had to go out and work. If I had an opportunity to move, I don't know if I would unless I could buy my own house. My father still lives in the same house in North Carolina that we were born in, and I do like an individual house. I hate living up five flights.

Living in a ghetto is . . . I can't really explain it to you. You . . . most people don't know what it is to be poor. I never wanted to be rich. I just wanted to have enough to live on. When King first got sick, I was so afraid because I didn't know what was going to happen to us. It's hard to tell the feel of hunger. When King got sick, all I had was two potatoes and some eggs, and I made an omelet for the children. That night I took him to the hospital, and they told me he would be there for a long time. I didn't know what to do. I came from a family where my father always provided. And yet, and still, I had a pride; when my husband got sick, I wouldn't ask my family for anything. They wouldn't have had too much to give because down South your salary's very low, and it takes most of what you make to survive on.

When he went to the hospital, Housing was after us for the rent, and I didn't know about social security. . .he was a veteran. I didn't know where to go—it was an awful feeling. My most comfort is my children and I used to sit up nights and hold the baby in my arms.

And another thing; when black men find things too tough for them, they either run away, or they start drinking, and then you live in fear. I used to hate to see Friday come because I wouldn't know whether he was coming home. I was lucky in one thing. I was never taught anything about birth control, but I didn't have my babies too close together, and I only had one miscarriage. So I didn't have that problem. In the meantime I used to work.

I used to do day work, and come home. I'd leave my children from one place to another. My oldest girl, when she got to be twelve, she said, "Mommy, I'll be really good if you just don't leave me no place." When the Antipoverty Program came, I worked with Head Start for about two years, and then I came to work for the Health Center. The reason I decided to work at the Center was that all these years I had left my children when I went to work, and now I could be close to them, if they called me I'd be right there.

I try to teach my children that it don't make no difference how much or how little you have if you enjoy what you do have, and we stick together as a family. I don't have any relatives here, only a sister-in-law. I don't care if it's black or white, if you're from the South they think you come from there to get something from somebody, and I always had a lot of pride. But I made some pretty good friends in the project; at nighttime when I had no food in the house, the neighbors came and brought me food.

The Health Center has been good to me. When Winnie was in the kindergarten in the morning class, I worked at the Center in the morning. When she changed over to the afternoon I did the same. After she'd been in school a year, I started working full time. The job has changed a bit since you left. Now they want to change us over to Social Service. I don't particularly like social workers or social work, but what I do like about my job is the closeness to people. In the ghetto we always saw social workers as people coming to ask us for papers. "You sign this, and you tell me that, and where is your insurance papers?" When King took sick, my house wasn't the best, but it was clean; the social worker that came wouldn't sit in my chair—she'd sit on the arm of the chair.

I tell this to our social workers at the Center. The Health Center has taught me more about people than any place I've ever lived. I've learned to respect social workers. I know that all social workers don't sit on your chairs' arms, and don't ask terrible questions, and they do understand how you feel.

I like the contact with people I work with, and the confidence some of the people have in me and the way they trust me. I understand that people have pride, and it's not lying when you're making extra money and you want to get ahead, and you don't tell them. Society's making us be that way. You're tired of the way life is.

I understand how people feel when they are caught off guard, and a nurse comes in when they've had a baby and their house isn't straightened up. Some days you just don't feel like combing your hair or getting up, but in the South you had to. If you didn't, the whites thought you were nothing, you were dirty. I know how some of them people feel because the same thing happened to me. And I tell them, if you're really tired and have too much to do, and I can get a homemaker for a few days to help you out, that doesn't mean you're a bad mother.

I've been helping out in two families from the South right now. One was a lady from Georgia. She had twelve children, and her husband just walked out on her. She tried to commit suicide quite a few times, but she's getting a little better now. There's another . . . a little girl from Alabama. She's had three sons and she's never married. One little boy had slight brain damage. She's really upset and cries a lot, because without a husband how can she survive in the ghetto with three little boys to care for? But she keeps a nice house for them; she's a mother; she's doing things for them.

Living in a ghetto and seeing people coming in there, it seems to me like the whole ghetto was a magnifying glass, and the whole world outside was looking at us like we was worms, and they was studying us. I've learned to accept the fact that people outside the ghetto don't understand *us,* but *I've* never been puzzled about people *outside* the ghetto. People outside think we are different.

Being black . . . are we any different than a person being white? We eat different but I can't see no distinctions in that. I felt the people who worked in the Clinic thought the black people in the project were different. They felt this special thing about the blacks, but I believe they think that if a white person lived here in the housing project, they chose to live there amongst us. I mean, they never looked at the fact that they was poor, and they had to live there too. I was reading a book one time, and it really made me angry because it said that black people's brains was smaller, and that's why they couldn't learn.

I've learned differently now about you and the Clinic, but when people first said to me about you, "Well, how can she care . . . she's white," I answered, "No, I don't know whether she cares or not." It took me time to be educated, to learn that you do care—it took time because we have been tricked a lot. The average black person is always looking for somebody to trick them, and it's hard to convince them that they're not being tricked.

People from the South had never been used to people thinking about them—about their health problems. I tell people I'm from the South myself and I know, for instance, how many days I went to school with a toothache. There was no dentist. I explain what the

Clinic is trying to do—to get the children examined early so they will have better health and good teeth. Another thing, you can kind of tell when a person don't want to be bothered with you that day. I told one lady from Mississippi (she had a terrible headache the day I came to visit), "I'll come back another day, you just tell me when." You should have seen her smile; she was so glad that somebody really cared.

As far as the Clinic, I think it's the most wonderful thing that has happened, but as far as the ghettos, I'd just like to tear half the buildings down and start again. But the Clinic has to be careful. It gets so bogged down with people with problems that it *can't* do anything about that sometimes it don't help people who should be helped. I mean people who have problems that can be helped, but they're too shy to come out and tell about it, and they're missed by the Center.

I think the biggest thing you can do is what you did for me by teaching me. We have attitudes that are not right either. I learned so much at the Clinic by changing my attitude to people— professional people, white people, Jews. I don't know why I resent Jews, but, when I was home, it was taught to me to resent it, I don't know why. We used to jump rope and I never thought about the word Jew—only from Christ was—you know. I used to jump rope and say, "If your father chews tobacco, then he's a dirty Jew." We used to say this all day, and there was one Jewish home, on the corner down there, and my mother'd say, "Oh, don't go in the Jew's house."

I don't know. I think it was just something that was put into us. When I came up here, everybody always said the Jews were cheating; that you couldn't trust them at all. But you see, when I started working, I worked with Jews. I was telling one Jew lady, she was a young girl, me and her were the same age, how we used to call Jews. Then I said, "I feel really bad, now I can understand why some white people hate a black person because they are also taught into these things." The people who have been nice to me are the Jews. When I went home I was telling my mother. I said, "Mom," I said, "How come?" Momma said, "I don't know." She said, "My mother taught us that."

Mrs. O'Reilly — Community Health Worker

Mrs. O'Reilly—thin, active, helpful, always on the run. A devout Catholic, Mrs. O'Reilly had a simple faith in God and a belief in the goodness of people. A good wife and mother, free of racism and religious prejudice, Mrs. O'Reilly found satisfaction in a life of service to those less fortunate than herself.

I think that the Health Center is one of the greatest things that really could come to a community. I've lived in the project for ten years, and I know how hard it was when mine were sick and you had to take them to East City Hospital, and if you brought them over to the baby clinic, they would tell you they were very sorry, but they couldn't take care of them because it was a well-baby clinic. And now to see . . . of course, my children are older now . . . but to see how the Center has come up and the many things we have now . . . we have the pediatrics . . . we also have emergency . . . upstairs now we have adult clinic. Since we've opened the census tracts, anyone can come, and we are now in the process of renovations, and when they are completed, we will have the whole second floor for adult services. Pediatrics on the first . . . adults on the second . . . and nursing on the third along with administrative. The entire community in the outside area has a chance to come down to our Center.

Of course, I realize there's been a lot of publicity about the Health Center and about the project in the newspapers and everything, but as a tenant, and living in the project amongst black people, I have found they are just like us. They're as human as we are, and I don't think that you can judge anyone, even in our own race, saying you're better than anyone, because we have good and bad in ours as well as they have in theirs. If you lived in a community like I've lived in and saw these people and their children . . . they have the same goals that we have, and they hope to reach them just like we do. And people claim they're frightened down there . . . I'm not any more frightened walking down there than I was walking up Main Street. I've never been threatened in the project.

I still work in the project, but I don't live there any more. I moved out three years ago. The reason I left is because I had a five room apartment with eight of us, and there wasn't any room, no closet space or anything. I was fortunate with six children to find this apartment. I have a duplex—one side, eight rooms, which is nice. One thing, when you live in the project, when you open the front door, you're right in the living room, which is very bad in the stormy weather. Or somebody comes in, they're right in your living room. But I can't say that I had any problems after living there for ten years.

We do have a drug problem, and that makes us a little more cautious. Like if I, for instance, were going out to work in the area, and I saw teenagers in the hall where I know they should be in school or working or something, then I certainly won't go by myself. I'd rather come back and ask someone to go with me, or check to see if they have a phone. But the Health Center has helped quite a few in the project that were on drugs and now are back on their feet and working, and hopefully they'll continue to stay that way. I think we have a drug problem in the whole city, and it's sad to think that outside the project they don't want to admit that there is a drug problem. Even up in my area where I live now, we lost three teenagers in one week from an O.D. . . . but yet these parents refuse to admit it. Whether it's the embarrassment or what it might be, it's very hard for a mother to say, "My son is on it." So I mean, it's just not the project that has a drug problem. I think it's everywhere, not just West Hill, everywhere. When you have teenagers, you really worry. I even worry about my twelve year-old because this is going on, and all my husband and I can do is just tell them, "I hope you know and understand . . . you've read the books . . . you've seen the pictures . . . just try to go straight." I find it so much harder trying to raise my children than it was for my parents raising us.

I think this generation has it much easier than we did growing up. And I think the parents are much more lenient with them. I think in a lot of cases, they get too much, and they're not as happy as we were. We didn't expect it because it just wasn't there, but today I really don't think that they value a dollar. The children expect a lot more from us than we did from our parents. And they're not as content as we were.

About myself, I've worked for the past five years as a neighborhood aide. I like it very much. I like to meet people, and it makes me feel real good if I go and I can help someone. I find that quite a rewarding job. I've worked with one family . . . she was very, very shy. She wouldn't talk only when you talked to her . . . asked her a question, and today if you saw her, you just wouldn't believe it. I mean, I was just astonished. Miss Ryerson runs this mothers' club where different mothers come and meet, and this woman in particular was very interested. Before, she was in her shell, and now she'll call up and she'll say, "I want to come to the meetings, and I want to be sure you're going to have it next week," and has really come way out, and it just makes me feel very good.

Right now, I think that my job is even more interesting. I have been working in the adult clinic, and it gives me a chance to meet different people and get some that aren't feeling too well. I'm still working outside, but I'm working like four hours a day in adult clinic, too. And if they're stuck, I work in mothers' clinic. And I'm getting many more nursing skills there. I enjoy that. I love people. Oh, I really do. I like meeting them. You find all kinds of problems, many problems. You can't solve them all. You say, "Well, I can't perform miracles or anything but I can help." And if they place their trust in you, even in a crisis they know they can get on the phone and call the Health Center, and there's always someone there that will be more than willing to help them. And I think that's the way it should be.

I think I'd really like to do nursing. I like nurses. If I were younger and given the opportunity. . .say five or six years. . .to go back and finish my high school and then go in, maybe I would train to be a nurse, but right now, with my family, my children and everything, I don't think I could. I'd be too tired. I have to work. I mean, if I wasn't working, it would be pretty rough, but I know my husband understands that, and we get along fine. I think we have a happy home life.

Sister Patricia is running a school, just starting now at the Health Center. She had four or five of us over this morning, and I think she can help us graduate, the ones that haven't graduated and the ones that want to go on. It's going to prepare us for the high school equivalency test. It's for anyone in the area who would be interested. She's been a great help to me. She's given me the books. I don't think I'd find it that hard getting a diploma.

Your book? You'll never be forgotten because you came down here and opened everyone's eyes, and everyone loved you. So I think you should put something about prejudice into that book. A lot of people that really don't understand just say, "Oh, I don't like the black, or the white." But really they should instill that there's good and bad in all, and that black people aren't bad. . .white people aren't bad. I don't think anyone's really bad. There's still a little good in every little bad. And I think if older people could look at a community like Bracken Field and stand watching little black children and little white children playing together, they would very seldom hear one say, "You're white," or "You're black." The little ones, they play and they're friends, and it's only in the homes that they're going to hear this, and then when they bring it outside, they're going to say, "Well, my mother don't want me to play with you 'cause you're black," or vice versa. And I think that's wrong. I think that in order to live together, we have to learn to get along together and to realize we all have a soul, and then it would be a better world to live in.

Mrs. Lane — A Community Worker

*With five young children to feed, no husband, and no day care, for
a period of three years Mrs. Lane left her children alone in bed in a
locked apartment each night and worked while they slept. Her
boisterous spirits, despite the circumstances, were never completely subdued, nor her vigorous likes and dislikes. Always fiercely
loyal to the Health Center, she strove upsparingly to exemplify the
Center's goal of service to the community.*

I come from a middle-class black family from the South. I was born
in South Carolina but raised in North Carolina by an aunt. My
mother died when I was a baby—I don't know her.

There were three classes of people down South where I lived,
non-professional, semi-professional and professional. I lived in the
professional group because my aunt's daughter was a teacher.
Nobody lived in my community but teachers, doctors, ministers.

I finished High School and wanted to be a social worker; my
cousin thought I should go to Teacher's College and then to Social
Work College. But my aunt was always so strict with me—she
wouldn't let me go out with the girls and boys—I ran away from
home and got married.

I was eighteen at the time, and I thought getting married and
having a baby would give me what I was looking for. I guess I felt
unloved. When my aunt found out about the marriage, I was
already pregnant. After I had my oldest child, I went to college for
a year, and then I got pregnant with the second child. I went back
to college again for another six months. My aunt was taking care of
me and the two children because my husband was young and unex-
perienced and couldn't really get a job. But after those six months
in College, my aunt said, "Well, okay, since you want to be grown
up, you just are going to stay home and take care of your own
babies."

So then we moved to Cleveland, but we didn't make a go of it
because my aunt had always done everything for me and the
children. I was ignorant of the facts of married life and how to do
things. My husband studied to be a mortician for a while, but then
he went into the Army during World War II, and after that we
separated, and I came to East City with the three children I had by
then.

Soon after I came to East City, I got pregnant a fourth time, and that was a turning point in my life. I really found out what hardship was all about. I had to go on Welfare but it didn't pay the kind of money it pays today. I was sick before Fanny was born— flat on my back.

Sadie was five or six years old at the time, Amos was older than her but a little limited, not retarded, but Sadie is very bright. I had a hot plate and the kids put it on a chair next to my bed, and I showed Sadie how to mix the flour and water and stuff to try and fix some food for them. I was sick, anemic, and I had falling out spells. The doctor told me to stay in bed. I had no strength, and by not getting the food I needed, I was just total weakness, you know.

I was living in a beautiful neighborhood. I was the only black that ever lived in that community; so therefore I was an outcast. Except for one white family that was nice to me and would take the babies and play with them.

Finally, after I had Fanny, one of my sisters separated from her husband and moved into Bracken Field, and I said, "Well, gee, I'll move in there too if you can get your light and gas and every- thing free." Another reason I moved was because the principal of the school told me about how a Jew family had moved into our community, and they had to move because the Irishmen wouldn't allow their children to play with the Jew children. The Jew family was really miserable; so the principal suggested I should move so my black children wouldn't come up with a conflict also. So I went to Family Service, and they got me into Bracken Field. But the pro- ject then, in 1954, was a beautiful place.

But now the whites started moving out, and all the blacks were moving in. You know, when we first moved in, it was all white; you could count the blacks on two hands. Then it started to get rough. As the whites left, they would bomb us. They would have gang fights—some of the children got burnt—that's how nasty and pre- judiced they were—they didn't want us in there. Even the principal of the school would tell our kids that they came from ghettoes and out of alleys; it was really tough for the kids to go to school.

I taught my children what a person say did not make them *be* that—it's up to each individual what you are. So your aims have to be high in order to get any place. I guess that's one advantage, liv- ing in the South, because we are taught if you don't want to be called "boy" you must go to school. Everything here in the North is whitewashed, and people is really fooled.

Meantime, when I moved into the project I was pregnant with Martin. I guess really the hardest part of my life was when I had five children, and I was getting nine dollars and eighteen cents every two weeks from Welfare. My husband was supposed to send me twenty-five dollars a week, and Fanny's father was supposed to give me eight dollars a week, but none of this money came in. So I went out and started working.

When CAP came along, I had just had a serious operation, but I got involved and was elected onto the CAP Board to help get it on its feet. Instead of keeping my appointment at the hospital, I was running to meetings in town, fighting to get CAP into Bracken Field. Most people in the community didn't want to say that they were poor—someone had to stand up and say "Yes, we are poor, and we need the money to help better our community." So it was myself and one or two others that really fought to get the money and started CAP here at Bracken Field. I know how hard the original people fought to get these things for Bracken Field. We even lost one of our members—an old lady who died right in the CAP office. But now I think CAP is one of the worst things that could happen to our community. It built a wall—people divided. They're only interested in the jobs and the money. I have no proof of this, but I believe that Bracken Field is getting more money than other projects, but we live more like pigs than anybody else. I feel it's because of our so called CAP representatives. They're not really representing the people; they're representing their pocketbooks.

I love people. I feel if I can set an example of first being at the top, and then getting down to the lowest any human can get with five kids and nine dollars and eighteen cents, and then gradually climbing back up, someone hopefully might say, "Look, Mrs. Lane made it—so can I." And then maybe another person will take after that person, and we will have a better community. But to have a better community, tenants have to be led to stand up and face facts and stop being brainwashed by the agencies in our community. When emergencies occur, where do they go? The Health Center. We *outreach* for health care at the Center. The community agencies should reach out to the people for other things.

I think the Health Center is one of the greatest things that ever happened. It's more like a family center, or friendly center. It plays a very major role here because the people there do more than see to health care. People feel free to call one of the community workers and tell them their problems, and the community worker relates back to the necessary person at the Center, and then they get help. I would prefer to see all the money that's going to the agencies all going to the Health Center so that we can have a bigger Center with more concerned people ready to stand up and say, "We are here to serve you."

Mrs. Martinez — Spanish Interpreter

When Mrs. Martinez escaped from Cuba, she and her group survived three days in a boat without food or water. Separated from her daughter, who remained in Cuba, Mrs. Martinez sought out her sister in East City. We employed her as the Spanish interpreter aide in the household census we conducted the first summer the center was funded, and later as interpreter aide at the Health Center. Mrs. Martinez loved everyone at the Health Center. Her soft heart and kindly nature, her generosity and willingness to help others without reservation, made her an easy target for exploitation in our tough neighborhood. But, somehow, this gentle lady to whom the affection of others was as necessary as food, managed not only to keep going, but to be a source of strength for a large number of her compatriots.

I was born in Cuba in the country. When I was born, I was very sick, and the doctor told my mother that she had to take me to Havana to see the doctors about my health—so I grow up in Havana. My father was a very nice man . . . he was a diplomat in Cuba for a period of forty years and my mother had a nice time when they got married. We have maids and gardeners. I was only seven years old when my mother died of TB. My father sent us to the best schools. I started the high school . . . went to the second year . . . I learnt to sew . . . to embroider . . . paint a little bit . . . a few things to make the life better. But from about 1935, everybody have a very hard time. Everything changed with the government. We was hungry for many days. But we survived.

I married when I was seventeen. My husband was nineteen. Yes, we were too young. My husband was working in a pier. He put on his shoulder big bags . . . five hundred pounds of potatoes . . . those heavy things. He was making good money, but he was too young. We was together ten years, and we have a daughter.

When I leave my husband, I have my own beauty parlor in my house, and I pay for my car, but then everything start to change again . . . with Castro . . . revolutions . . . Everything was different. So I tried to come to the United States, but I have nobody to bring me over here. I tried the first time to come over here with a doctor and his daughter and family. But when they tried to escape,

I can't reach the boat, and they was killed. The second time I can't reach the boat either, but the third time I made it and I escaped. So I'm here.

We brought fourteen children with us but my daughter wouldn't come. She's afraid of the water. She was nineteen, but she's afraid of water. I say, "You should come." She say, "No, no." I escaped myself. She also doesn't like flying. I don't know how she can come over here without flying. Or over the water in some way. I'm still waiting for her.

My sister was living in East City for nine years before I came here. But they moved to Miami soon after I came here. When I came to East City, I started to work in the apron factory. I'll never forget . . . I never worked in Cuba in a factory, you know. It was very hard for me to learn how to sew on the big sewing machine, the business machine. When I was supposed to move the machine front, I moved back. Too many times I break the needle, but I learned. About fourteen months I was working there, but I don't make good money. For me I have nothing. I have to make three hundred and eighty-eight aprons a day, for a dollar and twenty-five cents an hour. So I was working too hard.

After that I say, "No, I have to learn English because I have to go work some place else better than this." So I changed my job to electronics, and when I came back home, I'm going to the high school to learn English. I learn few English, and I start to feel better, and after I communicate with the person I feel happy, and I feel more happy now I can communicate more.

After I start to work in the electronic factory, I marry. But my husband start to drink, and everything went wrong. He has a lot of trouble because he drink and fight all the time. He was very nice before. So one day I was very, very sad. I went to the Employment Center in West Hill, and I ask them if I can go into the Peace Corps. They was very, very amazed that I want to ask for that kind of job. They ask me, "What for?" I said, "Because I going to go far away." I say, "I want to go some place I can help the people. I want to feel I can do something for somebody else." So they say, "Oh . . . we have a good job for you."

So I have an appointment to talk to Kate at the Health Center, and at first I was very sad, 'cause I think I'm going far away but East City was near. But soon I was very happy at the chance. So I find Kate and yourself, and I started to work with the household census in the whole area, asking the questions to the Spanish families . . . you remember? I tried very hard because I think it was good for me. So I almost have three years working for the Clinic now, and sometimes I'm upset . . . sometimes I'm blue . . . sometimes I'm happy, but I'm still here. I got so mad and so upset when you said you were going to leave us. Oh, I was crying. I cannot stay more in the meeting . . . I have to run down the stairs and cry by myself in a room over there in the Clinic.

I told you I was going to leave also, but you said I musn't leave because the Spanish families couldn't manage without me. Yes, too many of the Spanish families, they come to my place to get their hair done and because they know me they come to the Clinic. I think they trust me . . . whatever they tell me I tell the doctors, and they are sure I translate for her in the best way I know to the doctors. We have not only the Cuban people, but also from Colombia and from the different Spanish countries. They are very poor. We have families from Panama, Columbia, Ecuador, the Dominican Republic, and now they start to come from Portugal. The most we have is from Cuba and Puerto Rico.

Many Spanish families live in West Hill in the area of the Clinic. They have lots of problems. As soon as they come to this country, they go to Welfare because they need help. They help them, but they has to wait too long until they have furniture. Like this week at the Health Center, we have two families from Cuba that have been here almost three months, and they are still waiting for the furnitures, and they are sleeping on the floor. Some neighbors give them mattress or blankets.

You would be surprised. Some of the social workers at the Health Center and all the nurses are learning Spanish with Mr. Gonzales, like I was doing before, but now I have no time because I am too busy all the time. Everybody's learning Spanish, the doctors also. Yes, we have good doctors at the Health Center.

Some of the families have a hard time. Like Mrs. Lopez. Her neighbors wasn't very good with her. The poor lady, she was almost crazy. Her husband was beaten very bad. All his head was smashed and wounded. He was just like paralyzed. They say the Puerto Rican people hated him. I don't know why. The poor lady was suffering a long time, and at last she had a nervous breakdown. Some time ago she moved away from the neighbors—to another part of the city.

Do you remember Mrs. Guevara? She has twins now, a boy and a girl. She has a lot of trouble also. She send her boy, five years old, to the supermarket. A colored boy tried to take away his money, so he pushed him. A gang came to Mrs. Guevara's house to break the windows and break the door. They beat the husband and the little boy because he pushed the colored boy, and Mrs. Guevara doesn't know what it's all about; so she was very afraid. Then she has the babies, the twins, and they was very sick with diarrheas and fever, and they were very, very tiny. So we start to take care of that trouble like we always do in the Clinic . . . help the people, and she finally moved from that place, into the project.

There was trouble between black people and Puerto Rican people. I don't know why. But the Cuban people not have trouble with colored people. The Puerto Rican people say the colored people hate them. We know also a few Puerto Ricans hate the Cuban people. I don't know why. They say too many Cuban people go to Puerto Rico, and they take their place—build a business. I don't know why not because if they live over there and have a place to make a business, why not? They don't push anybody. The Puerto Rican people call the colored people all kinds of names they don't like. They call them "mojetos." Mojetos is the . . . like you say . . . black people but in bad words, you know, like "nigger." The first time when they say to me the "mojetos" I say, "Who is the mojetos?" And she tell me, "Well that is the colored people here."

I say, "Why do you call that?"

They say, "Because we call the colored people that a long time ago."

We can have a place for everybody. I don't know why we don't love each other. We would have better life, and we can live better. I don't know why people fight. Myself I don't hate anybody. In Cuba the blood are mixed up, you know, white-black, so we don't make no difference . . . we don't see the difference.

I'm getting along great with everybody in the Clinic. But do you remember the first time Dr. Mbayo came to the Health Center? Oh . . . I had a very bad time with him. I remember I say his name wrong because I don't know how to say it. I call him I think a different name. So he stop me—it was his first day he work here. He say, "Mrs. Martinez, you have to say my name right." Oh I was surprised, you know, I was shocked. I say, "Oh yes, would you please let me know how you say your name, and maybe I can say it better." He don't tell me. He write it down on paper, and he give it to me, and he say, "Show everybody how to say my name." But he don't tell me how I have to say. So I still say the same. I tell everybody, "This is the new doctor from Biafra; he doesn't want anybody to say his name wrong; so we have to learn to say it." So Mrs. Pederson and I were telling two or three times his name till I had to come back to him to translate for Spanish people, and when I got to say "Dr. Mbayo," I say it wrong again. And he stop me again and he say, "That is not my name. You have to learn to say my name. Will you please, Mrs. Martinez?" And I say, "Yes, Doctor, I will try." Oh, he give me a bad time. You know, I wasn't mad with him. I was mad with myself because I can't say it. But in the end, when he go, we were sad, because he was very nice doctor truly.

Mrs. Pederson and I have been working together for almost two years in the Clinic. I feel like she is part of my family. We also go on our vacations together. We can't go this year. We got no money. But the Clinic is changing. We have new staff . . . new people come and go. And that's hard for me. I feel everybody's my family . . . see all the time I feel that way. If I meet you today, I don't feel that I meet you today. I feel that I meet you a long time ago. I'm that way, so as soon as they go away, I feel, "Oh my goodness, everything's wrong . . . why the people have to go?" I know they have to change jobs. They may be going to some better place, or they may want to change, but I don't want it. I'm learning now how to feel different. Like the same Cuban families I know for a long time now, they say I'm no more Spanish because I feel more like the American people. I know everything's changing in me, but I still loving everybody. I learning to wait until people come to be friendly to myself. But when they go and I can't see them no more, I feel everything is breaking inside.

The Spanish people are not involved with community things. When they come to the Clinic we ask them if they have appointment; they sit down and they stay. They are not involved with things around. They go to work, or raise the family, keep the house, send the kids to school, that's all.

The Spanish people always call me for help. At my home . . . two o'clock in the morning . . . three o'clock . . . the ladies . . . they going to have the baby . . . they can't call the police . . . they call me. "Please Juanita . . . Mrs. Martinez," see they are my friends, . . . they call me "Juanita, Please Nana," . . . they call me Nana sometimes like the grandmother . . . "Call the police, I'm going to have the baby." So at that time I call the police. My telephone is a business telephone. It's like an agency. But I enjoy.

Alice Gray—Clinic Worker

Alice Gray came from a family of fifteen children. She was brought up "very religious" by strict parents. After her marriage broke up, she moved into the project with her four children. Mrs. Gray was an immaculate housekeeper. A reserved woman, she worked hard for the education and betterment of her children. She didn't believe in spoonfeeding people and thought the Health Center staff were often too permissive in their attitudes. Direct in her approach, unafraid to voice her opinions, Mrs. Gray made us think hard about certain items of health care practice we had all taken for granted. Who, if anyone, has the right to knock on patients' doors is one of the troublesome areas we never fully resolved.

In a community like the housing project, you have to know exactly which way you're going, and you have to give your kids a kind of strength, backbone, that they really need . . . more than I think any place else. If they want anything out of life, they're going to have to work hard for it, and the best thing in the world is to get all the education they can possibly get because there just isn't any room for dummies, and this is exactly how I explain it to them.

Do you know how I got my job at the Health Center? Mrs. MacGregor (who was working for you on the statistics) came by my house when she was taking the census, and after she had finished, she wanted to know if I wanted to ask her a question. I said, "Yes, tell me how do you go about getting a job at the Health Center?" And that's how I became an aide. I say, you can't sit back and hold your mouth shut.

My husband and I are separated now. I support the children. Before I worked for the Health Center, I used to work at the switchboard at the Talmadge Hotel and after that in a department store. Then I worked in a meat department . . . I've learned almost every job I can think of.

There's not too many people I talk to—I don't consider too many people even friends. I live rather close to myself, because I have a certain kind of respect and certain kind of dignity. I don't have people running in and out of my house because this I don't like. I'd do anything in the world I possibly can do if you need help, as long as it's outside my door. And I don't like rowdiness . . . I don't like loudness . . . and I like to be respected 'cause I'm going to treat other people with respect, so, therefore I say, "You don't get no more out of life than you put into it." So these are the things that I instill within my kids; these are my rules that I live by, and I'm pretty comfortable living with them.

I don't like to get in race things either. I try not to be a racist, but this race business more and more is coming up, and you know because you are black, you're going to have twice as hard a time getting what you want as anybody else. When I hear about all this black power stuff, I say, "Gee, I never needed anybody to wake me up to the fact that I had to be proud of my blackness . . . I've always been proud of it." I've been pretty proud of me, too, because I guess this is how my people brought me up.

This is one thing *you* can feel proud of, one thing people say, and you hear this all over West Hill—the best thing ever happened to West Hill is the Health Center. Regardless of all of its shortcomings, if you're looking for security . . . like looking for somewhere to hide and you don't know where to go, the Health Center is it . . . regardless of what your problems is, there's always somebody there you can turn to. The people would like to see the Health Center go into a much broader field of health . . . they would like to be able to see as complete a medical center as possible—not just pediatrics and obstetrics—they want a twenty-four hour service, both medical and dental.

We poor folks have always gotten everything second-handed. I say, "Why can't we get a decent place set up and make the people take care of it?" You've got nurses going around trying to teach people cleanliness, if you can't give it to them in their homes, what's a better way of starting out with than the Center . . . show them that this is a Center . . . this is for you . . . this is for you to take care of . . . it's yours. If you can get people to start thinking that this is mine, and we want to keep it because this is the only thing we got . . . it's something you can impress upon them. We have put this here, now it's up to you to take care of it, and if they would do that, I think they would be a whole lot better off. But I think there's been too much leniency on many people's parts, trying to please people and do everything you think people want you to do, and you wind up getting nowhere.

And another thing, nursing has put itself out to the point of making appointments for people, bringing people in . . . forcing the aides to be babysitters, and this is something the aides never liked. I figured I had kids of my own, and nobody ever baby-sat for me

. . . I had to pay a babysitter. And especially when you know people will leave their kids home nights to go to what they want to do in the evenings; but yet, and still, when it comes time to bring their child to the Clinic, they can't do it. They give you all the excuses. "I've got so many children . . . I've got to get this one dressed . . . I've got to get that one dressed." So get them dressed. After you have done everything you can, Doctor, there are some people you have to let go, and it might sometimes break your heart to do so, but you have to let go and put that person on their own. As long as some people know that they've always got somebody to depend on to throw their problems on . . . they will do it, and so, therefore, instead of making people independent, we make people dependent. I think the rules in the Health Center need to be a little more strict. I don't say that they have to be so strict that people are afraid to breathe, but I do think that there has to be some kind of stricter standards.

At the staff conference last week, we sat down and talked as a group about the goals of the Clinic, and I'm pretty sure that we all had the same goals in mind. The first was to give medical care. Then we could start thinking about adding all these other things together . . . getting involved in community activities . . . housing . . . and all these things, but health came first. The problem is how do you go about getting medical care? Should we continue to go out knocking on peoples' doors and persuading them?

We came to the conclusion in certain instances we have been pampering the community too much. I always believe you're going to get that few who are going to constantly be there regardless of whether they need it or not. Then, too, we spoke about how much confidence the community has in us. It had been said that people in the community was out talking about patients who had come to the Clinic. So this was another thing to come up. Do people feel we're prying when we visit their homes? Well, I always thought that aides had been used somewhat as peeping toms for nurses and for Social Service—in other words they almost expect them to be some kind of an information bureau for their use. I understand Social Service had gone out into people's homes and asked all these personal questions. I say, "Don't force yourself on anybody."

I think people should be *invited* into homes. If I was a social worker or if I had to go into a person's home because they needed help or they had been referred to me, then I would go into that person's home and say this to them: "I'm not here to snoop or pry into your affairs; I'm a social worker," and explain the functions of my job. "Now I'm here to help if you want to be helped, but if not, then, you know, this is up to you, but I want you to know I'm here just in case." I would leave it just like that and then just sit back and wait, and I think you'll get much more out of people than you would by going there asking them this.

Employing more community people at the Center? Community people—I think they're good in certain jobs, like my job. I feel very comfortable in it because I don't have to get that close to people—I don't have to really get involved in other people's affairs. Like these team meetings we have. I wouldn't want to be in one of those team meetings because, see, these people I live with. I constantly see them. Okay, I don't think they'd feel very comfortable with me, knowing that I might know something about them. When they see me on the street, they say, "Hi, Mrs. Gray," and I can ask them about one of their kids—about themselves, and that's it. I think it's much better to have people who don't live so close . . . like yourself . . . who live away from the place. I wouldn't say necessarily away from the problems because I wish in a way that you could be with the problems—I mean there are different opinions about this, you see? Maybe if a person who was a professional could give us a program to be assistants to social service or social service aide or something like this, and they really thought that the community could accept this, then train these people and let them go into the homes and let them talk and feel people out.

Mrs. Taylor—A Motherly Clinic Worker

Mrs. Taylor had lived in the housing project almost twenty years when I began to work at the Health Center. We placed her in the reception area to welcome patients, many of whom she knew. Pleasant and equable in temperament, Mrs. Taylor would often be soothing a baby while the mother was being examined, and generally she eased the process of receiving medical care. I called her the "clinic grandmother"—a role she fulfilled admirably.

I finished High School at East City Girls Trade School. That's where I took my arts and sewing. I always wanted to be a teacher. A sixth grade teacher . . . I don't know why but I thought that was the most fascinating class. My teacher didn't particularly like me; so she didn't make my life very happy, but I liked the sixth grade.

I was very spoiled as a child. My sister of eighteen was killed when I was three years old. It was her first job. She was working the elevator, and she stepped out to see if anyone was coming, and the elevator went up, and she fell into the pit. She had been an accomplished pianist and dressmaker, and everything that she did my mother fussed over me to do. When I got married, my husband sort of spoiled me too.

He cooked and he cleaned. He was very good. I believe in housewifely duties, but I'm not a great housekeeper. I don't go wild buying sheets and curtains. I can pass by these things as long as I can find a book department. He treated me like a little girl, called me Missy till the babies came, and then I was mother. He had a son of seventeen before he married me, and he was a marvelous father. He loved my mother too. If he had stayed on, I would have been even more spoiled because he was marvelous. But he just wasn't responsible. He had that irresponsible Cherokee Indian way, you know, they got to go and take off. And then he just sort of fell by the wayside. He had ulcers, and he took some kind of dope or something that deteriorated him because after a while he was gone, and that was that. I didn't go running out trying to find him and neglecting the children. I figured he was a man, he could take care of himself. It was up to me to take care of the children. And if he had ever wanted to come back, the door was open. Now that I know a little bit more about medicine, and dope and things like that, maybe I would have been able to help him. He was a very good husband, and I'm grateful for what he taught me, but I was sort of grass widow for fourteen years. He died a few years ago, so now I'm a full fledged widow. I guess I raised the kids pretty good.

After he left me, around 1953, I moved into the project. I was on Aid for Families of Dependent Children. I knew West Hill pretty well, and I knew some of the families that had moved into the project. It was sort of friendly, and the children got along fine. My mother and father moved in a few years after I did. She was going blind with glaucoma and cataracts. As the boys got older, it was getting a bit rough, and the boys were getting into a bit more trouble, especially Jim. I'd be down in the office half the time getting him out of scrapes. Jim is a playboy. He doesn't have ambition. Without Jim there'd be no need for prayers, lighting candles in church or rosaries at night. He says when the summer is over he may go in the Navy. I try not to worry about them. I try not to push them or nag them. Both boys were in the service, and Billy was in Vietnam. My daughter, Rochelle, married a very nice Puerto Rican boy. They live in the same block I do.

When my mother died, my father moved in with me. It's always been a dream of mine to keep my family together. I've always wanted to have one of those ideal things like the big house up on the hill with mother in the middle and all the children living around. I don't like this thing of being spread all over the place and calling up people.

The project did change from the time I first moved in. It used to be cozy. We had good times, and we'd spend a lot of time out in the hall talking. Our doors were open. Most of the children in my building have grown up there since babies. But the newer people that came up, I don't know where they come from, but they don't seem to have the same attitude as the people who have grown up with my children. They don't seem to have any respect for their parents, let alone anybody else. Some of the mothers yell at the children so viciously I don't see how the children could want to have respect for them, and most of the mothers are so young I don't think they know much about enjoying their children anyway.

Then there's this racial business. When the civil rights started, this racial movement started coming in here. The CAP people were very nice, but they wanted everybody to be black that worked there. The Puerto Ricans keep pretty much to themselves in little family groups. They don't like the Cubans. The Cubans are more socially minded in a way than the Puerto Ricans. They are the middle class Spanish that came here . . . doctors and lawyers and things like that. They're the ones that will probably build up the Spanish community.

You want to know how I started with the Health Center? Well, when it was just a well-baby unit in the neighborhood hall, they wanted someone that could come in two days a week to keep the children who kept going up on the stage from falling off, and keeping them quiet because the doctors couldn't hear anything. They didn't have cubicles then; it was just wide open and very noisy. If Dr. Bach thought a child had a heart murmur, she had to take the child into the kitchen outside and shut the door so she could hear! They just wanted to have a play lady.

By that time my children were all in school, so I went down. We got coloring books together and crayons and magazines, and we got a little area as far away as we could and the children liked it. Once when they were kind of short-handed, the Public Health nurse showed me how to weigh the babies. So I started helping with that, and I just kept on. And it got more interesting.

My social worker was kind of angry with me. The social workers really wanted you to go out and work for money, and I was there at the Neighborhood House all day Tuesday, and on Monday I'd stay on after Clinic for Arts and Crafts and Girl Scouts. I also did some tutoring. She'd say, "Well, if you can be there you could be working." But I had no intentions of working. My mother wasn't young when she moved to the project, and she began failing much more at this time. When she was sick, I could be within running distance of getting to her. I just wouldn't give in to my social worker. I told her, "What can I bring home for the children better than the people that I meet at work? I don't meet people of that kind in factories. I meet doctors from all over the world. I intend to stay, and I won't go downtown where I can't get home at a moment's notice." I really enjoyed fighting with the social workers because I never asked them for anything. I took my money as it came and used it. I wasn't always running down asking for something extra—I got along on what I had.

The Health Center moved over to the housing apartments about 1965, and in 1967 I went on payroll and went on full time work. By that time Rochelle was seventeen and would soon be eighteen, and that would be the end of AFDC. I really enjoy my work because I really feel as though we're helping, and we're not

afraid to say something to the doctor. We have a baby . . . she's
about three months old . . . she has a secretion . . . I call it to the
doctor's attention. They take a culture. It may not be anything, but
I don't feel, "Should I say something?" I tell the doctor immediately, and it makes you feel more a part of the Clinic. You really have the right to help these people.

I think the people have benefited by the Health Center and that
they really like the fact that they can go to a community place
where they get the same thing as in the hospitals, especially for the
children. And the adults . . . they really are so happy that they can
come to the Health Center. They are like children—they come
bouncing in. It would be very nice if you would write how it grew,
and what kind of people you work with, and what kind of people
live in the housing project.

People really use the Center. Sometimes it looks ridiculous
. . . all the people coming in . . . such little things that probably
could be done at home, perhaps, but they come in, and they'll wait,
and they don't get too upset if they have to wait too long . . . very
few will go stamping out. I think it's got a lot to do with our doctors. They are so wonderful.

The difference between the Health Center and an ordinary
clinic? The atmosphere for one thing. It's a friendly atmosphere.
We always try to talk to everybody . . . we know them a little more
intimately than they would in a regular hospital clinic. I think we
have a lot more fun with the doctors too—there's not too much pro-
tocol. A lot of people when they first come they just can't understand it, especially when they come from another country. At
first they don't understand our silly American ways, but it's just
the way we are. I don't think we're trying to put on an act for
anybody. We just love all these kids. We get mad with them
sometimes. We have some that come in screeching. It looks like
hell. We say the day is complete here. We're just natural I guess.
It's not put on. We just enjoy seeing people.

I'd like to see the Clinic grow. Not just health, but maybe
some culture for these people. If the housing project is fixed up,
many people will feel better about living in it. It's so run down . . .
some of the places look like a disaster area. Many of the people
come to us for help more to talk than for medical problems. We
don't want to seem nosy, but anyone who comes in that needs help
we try to find out how we can help. It makes you feel good if you're
helping somebody.

Mrs. Morrison From South Carolina—
A Social Work Assistant

Mrs. Morrison graduated from high school in the South and is attending college courses at night, while working at the Health Center. Over the years she has attended courses in mathematics, sociology, anthropology and psychology. Her husband, a cook, wants to return to the South and open a restaurant, but Lisa, their daughter, is at boarding school in a suburb of East City, and Mrs. Morrison feels that Lisa's education is paramount. She gets great satisfaction from her job and is much respected by the Health Center staff and community for her ability and compassion in its performance.

I was born in a small town in South Carolina, and I guess you might say I had some advantages. My father and mother bought the home that mother still lives in when I was seven. It's a beautiful place. We lived right in the city—we couldn't raise cattle like you could in the country, but my father always had enough room in the backyard to keep chickens, and he had a little space for his garden. It was nice because we had fresh tomatoes, okra, corn, just in that little space, two rows of everything.

Helping people, I guess, more or less came natural to me because I remember as a child, I would see my father work at a bank all day, and go sit with a sick friend all night. And I've always known my mother to help people because when I was coming up, she was a home economics teacher. She also had an adult class in the evening, and I don't think she had a scarf or a pillowcase or anything that didn't have some kind of fancy work on it. I can remember them both helping people, and when my daughter started going to school, I just got out in the community and started helping people also.

That wasn't what I started out to do though. I had started taking piano lessons. When I was nineteen, I came to East City to go to the Conservatory of Music but I just didn't go. I wanted to study at the Conservatory, but I got to East City in December, and I was going to apply to the Conservatory the following September. In the meantime I got a job, and soon after that I got married.

I became an upholsterer. I was the first woman upholsterer the shop hired. I stayed at the shop for years, but when I became pregnant, I left and didn't go back to work again until Lisa was about nine years old.

When Lisa got to that age, after I'd got her to school and cleaned the house, I'd have nothing to do. It got boring. I was living in the Garden Park Housing Project, and there were a lot of elderly people living there, and I'd help them. It started with my friend Sarah's mother who was visiting her from Durham, North Carolina. In those days there were no organizations like Mothers for Adequate Welfare, you know, all these organizations that fight for people. Sarah's mother was sick, and she took her to one of the big hospitals in East City. They gave her mother a hard time there because she was visiting, and Sarah was on Public Assistance. I got very angry about it, and I took her mother back to the hospital myself and had it out with them. Anyhow they saw her, and she was taken care of.

I got interested in housing because I was living in a housing project myself. I still am. I wanted to see things go better, so I joined with a few others and we got a steering committee going. Then we started the first Tenant's Association in East City (T.A.C.). My job was to organize the tenants to update and better where they lived. We fought for better police protection, foot-patrolmen, cleaner areas and the usual things that people fight for.

At that time the manager, Mr. Owens, was having a lot of problems with certain tenants, and he asked me if I would give him a hand and go and talk to them. It worked out very well. Some tenants were having quite a bit of problems with the police, but I made myself known to Station 9, and I seemed to have a very good success with the police. I've always been known to have a big mouth! It got to the point where people instead of calling the police would call me, and I'd call the police. So whenever people would see me in Garden Park—it was kind of a joke—they'd go get a box and put it down—''She's going to get on her soap box now.''

I was the first president of the Tenants' Association, too, and we were the first to have kids from the outside coming in to clean the project. We've been first in a lot of things where projects are concerned. We raised tomatoes, though we were told nothing would ever grow. They would take pictures of our flower gardens over there. And we were pretty proud of our development. We were doing good. Mr. Owens was a good manager. He would stay long hours, and he took an interest in the place, not just collecting the rents. He had compassion, people liked him, and I guess every-one wanted to please him, so we had a really nice development.

Then I went to school. I did a business course and learned all about office machines, typing, secretarial work, everything except shorthand. The Head Start program had just started, and I became a teacher's aide. But my father died at this time, and I had to go back South for six weeks. When I came back, I worked as a receptionist at the Day Care Center. I didn't really like it—I never cared for office work—it's too confining. But I stayed with it until I got a call from Family Service to tell me about a new government project called Project Enable. I finished that course on a Tuesday, and on the Wednesday I went to work for the Health Center.

The job I'm doing—community worker with the Social Service Department of the Health Center—I like. I would do it for money or without money. At the time I first started getting into that kind of work, there was nothing like the War on Poverty, and OEO; I did it because it made me feel good to do it. When the War on Poverty first began, and all the guidelines and everything was coming out of Washington, I can remember on Sundays we would all canvass the streets putting out pamphlets, putting up posters, letting everybody know long before the money actually came. And when they had to have a twenty-man community board in all the areas, we worked . . . we worked . . . and set up all that.

My job at the Health Center is helping people. In the course of a day, I deal with many different problems. Take one case I saw yesterday. The girl is eighteen years old and pregnant. Her family hasn't been told. Her parents live in the South, but she has a sister and several brothers. My job in this case was simply a matter of breaking the news to the family—to ease it as best I could, so that they wouldn't jump on her or make her feel worse than she already does. Or sometimes my job is fighting the Welfare Department to help a family that is not getting sufficient money, or sometimes it's taking people out to get estimates for furniture. See—if a family is on public assistance, they're entitled to furniture. For years it's been known that a family on public assistance shopping for furniture automatically gets shown the worst, even after the law was passed that they could get new furniture. And even though they're allowed new furniture now, a lot of people don't know enough about it. If it looks good they buy it, and three months later it's broken. It doesn't have to be fancy, but it should be strong. I've found a very good warehouse type place in Old Town where the owner knows the welfare guidelines, offers people choices, and gives good furniture for reasonable prices.

My main function is finding housing for people. Shortly after I came to work at the Health Center, I worked with a family where the mother was seven months pregnant and they hadn't had running water in five months. The woman had to carry water up five flights of stairs to flush the toilet. This was in East City and only about three years ago! The building was owned by a church! I had to go to the Housing Inspection Department who took the landlord to court. I managed to get that family moved into Bracken Field. Anything to do with housing is basically my job. I want to see everybody with at least a roof over their heads.

Projects aren't the best places to live, but it's not because of the building. Those buildings are just as strong and built just as good as any of your high-rise apartments that's going up now. The difference is the price you pay. You pay maybe three hundred or four hundred dollars a month for a three or four-room apartment in a high-rise. If the people in the project paid that kind of money, they'd get twenty-four hours maintenance and security services. Since there's a maximum rent that you pay in the project, and since some people pay as little as thirty dollars a month for rent, they don't get these things. The difference is in the upkeep. Because there's no proper maintenance and security, there's vandalism.

Why do I think poor people dislike social workers? The new welfare workers now are for the people, but the workers that have been in there ten, fifteen, twenty years acted as though the money was theirs, and it was coming out of their pockets. Maybe it was a policy that the less you gave a family, the better it was for the welfare worker—I couldn't say. Certainly, people weren't treated as people; they were a case, a number. The welfare workers looked down on them. And years ago they would come in and search your home, you know, look in your closets, and God forbid if you had a man's shoes there or something.

Everything depended on the worker, and if she was out to get you, there was nothing you could do. One social worker in Garden Park would come by early in the morning, say seven o'clock, and knock on your door to catch you. People in Garden Park got so sick of it, they beat her up, and she went to work some place else. You couldn't get what the law entitled you to—if your worker said you got it, you got it. But all that's changed the last few years. You know about certain things you're entitled to now, regardless of what the worker might say, like a pregnancy allowance and a layette. Also you can be living with your husband and still be entitled to a supplement. Some of the change came about when welfare elevated their standards for their employees. Of course, some of the workers from the old days are still employed, but the new ones are different—some of them have even gone on strike.

Sister Patricia, A Religious—
A Witness to the Celebration of Life

Sister Patricia, young, serene and pretty, is one of a growing number of young religious men and women active in the new reform movement of the Roman Catholic Church.

Before she came to work in the Health Center as a social worker, she had worked and lived in a psychiatric hospital sharing the life of these "outcasts." She had worked and lived also in children's institutions with children who had been neglected or abandoned by their patients. But these experiences were with specialized, isolated communities removed from the mainstream of American culture. Living in the Bracken Field community was an entirely new experience for her.

When I took the job as social worker at the Health Center, I came to live in the housing project. I am a Sister of the religious order of St. Vincent de Paul. St. Vincent's rules were that the nun's cloister should be the streets of the city and the wards of the hospital, and her only veil that of modesty, her cell a rented room.

So it became a tradition to be a witness to the fact that people do have a value whether they're wealthy or poor, educated or uneducated. Their worth has to be witnessed not only in word but in deed, which is a very old tradition in the Judeo-Christian tradition. So from the beginning there are records of Sisters going to feed the galley slaves, nursing the sick in their own homes, going into the streets. Of course, times change, and even within our own religious community, it became difficult to sell the idea that we should live this way again. It isn't much accepted. But there's a new movement in the Church—less a revolution than a reform movement, a returning to the original religious inspiration but adapted to modern culture.

So this is the background to my coming into a poverty area and living the life I do. It's a kind of return to an age-old tradition. Many of the orders of religious women, in this country particularly, are doing what I'm doing. I think there are probably small groups of nuns living in almost all housing projects in East City. But it's difficult and not accepted by some Catholics.

I've been a nun for about ten years. I received my Masters in Social Work in New York City before entering the order and lived and worked in the slums for quite a while. So I have had the experience of working in poor areas just as a professional. I must say I certainly have a different outlook now than I did then. At the time I graduated, I recall being very much impressed with Dorothy Day, who is a pacifist in the Catholic Worker movement. Her feeling was that too often professionals are only interested in what they can do *for* a person, how they can improve him or solve his problems; they aren't interested in the person himself regardless of whether he can solve his problems or not.

My initial impression in coming to live here was the tremendous variety and vitality of the people and their ability to celebrate life, a certain affirmation that life is worth celebrating despite its difficulties. The second thing that impressed me was the reaction of the people who lived outside the project to those who lived in it. They couldn't believe that Sister Mary and I lived here and were still alive. They constantly told us how bad it was here, almost as if it was a battleground.

The people outside the project are mostly white, of course, and the people in the project predominatly black, but those who live outside don't identify with the white families of the project either. They are mostly working class people, many fairly recent immigrants from Ireland, still with a brogue; others may have been here thirty or forty years, pinched pennies and saved and bought their own little houses. And now they see it all threatened; the neighborhood, they say, is going down, and they have cut themselves off completely from the project and from the Spanish speaking people moving in around them.

When we first moved in, we thought that maintenance was the biggest problem but now we think the biggest problem is lack of protection. We felt at first that we shouldn't be afraid because that would somehow show weakness, but I think living here, we have slowly picked up the project peoples' own fears and cautions. This isn't particularly a racial thing, but it's a matter of crime and violence.

We used to think of poverty as a lack of clothes, a lack of food, but now, as a witness to poverty, we almost have to share something else. We are all victims of crime and violence and have a certain helplessness to do anything about it. I think this is probably *the* problem of poverty; being poor is living in a poor neighborhood. You may have a little more money than somebody else living in a better neighborhood, but because of prejudice or some other reason, you can't move into a neighborhood where there is less crime and better police protection. So how much money you have doesn't indicate how much of a victim you're going to be according to my definition of poverty. And you have to adjust to taking precautions.

The community has taught us; they've been very good to us. I think they see it as their duty to take care of us. I think, too, as Sisters we have been better accepted because our motives are not questioned. They know we aren't going to take money, and we aren't going to study them as objects; they feel that everybody else has not paid much attention to them—the churches have not paid much attention to them either. So now they feel they have certain obligations to take care of us rather than that we are going to come in and do something for them. It's been important that they have been able to do something for us, to protect us.

I live with Sister Mary, who is a teacher. Stella Jones and the Health Advisory Group gave us advice and helped us get a very centrally located apartment on a more main thoroughfare on the fourth floor. On a main thoroughfare there's less activity, fewer places to hide. They also told us what kind of lock to put on the door, not to let people in, to get an unlisted number.

We usually don't go out alone at night, since last fall, when Sister Mary was mugged coming up our stairs on her way back from work. It was getting dark early, and it was Friday which is a bad day because it's payday. We were advised not to carry purses and to carry our money hidden, but the kids have gotten wise to that—they rip off the coat to see where the money is hidden. She said she wasn't afraid of the two teenagers because she knew they didn't want to hurt her; all they were after was her money, and they wanted to get it quickly. They had to rip off her coat and knock her down, rip off the pocket where she had the car keys and the apartment keys. We immediately called the police, but they didn't come. I remember we called again and explained to the Irish cop that we were Roman Catholic nuns, thinking this would certainly make them come, but it didn't. I remember having this feeling that they really didn't care.

Then we called one of the neighbors. Mr. Donnelly came over and shortly there were five or six people gathered to help. One of the men took the coil out of the car so it couldn't be stolen. Somebody else made sure the superintendent came out to change the security lock so that the kids couldn't come back and strip the apartment. They were very concerned that one of us had been robbed. At that time we were wearing very ordinary clothes, nothing that would signify we were nuns. Now, particularly if it's after five, and if we're in an area where we are probably not known, we have a veil that we can put on and take off very easily.

You also have the feeling that it's one thing to have a pickpocket or somebody take money—but a physical assault, the psychological impact of this is an added kind of violence to the human being, which certainly most of the elderly here have experienced. The black women are very much afraid to go out, too— the younger ones particularly talk about how frightened they are. They stay in after dark. This is the way of life.

The other thing you feel is that if the crimes were committed by people outside the project, the whole community could be united against this outside force, but there's this terrible feeling that it might be their own teenagers doing it, or their next door neighbors, or their good friend's teenagers. This is what splits the community apart; people are fearful of each other, of working together, not just wanting to get out of the project.

A large proportion of crime is due to drugs but not completely. There are a lot of twelve or thirteen year-olds who are mugging and burglarizing because it is such an easy way to make money. The value American society places on money certainly encourages this sort of thing, and the switchover from making money for an honest day's work to making money by playing the stock market, or making money by a hustle (which is the equivalent of playing the stock market where we live) isn't so different. People just have to find a different form to beat the system. I think they feel that to have money is to have self-respect, particularly for the boys, a way of demonstrating their manhood.

And another thing, the kids look at the best dressed fellows around and the ones who have the biggest cars and see that they're the ones who are the drug pushers. But you can't blame it all on drugs. The boys see that the men who've stayed with their families in the project, gone out to work every day, maybe held down two jobs, don't have big cars. But the boyfriends who aren't paying for any family, who don't assume responsibility for children they may have, these are the men who have money left over to buy a car. The boys see so many mother-based homes. I think there's a great deal of concern among the women about their men, and about their sons particularly.

When you have lived here for a while without a car, you learn how difficult it is to get around. When you see the loneliness of a mother whose kids have no father, you begin to understand why women on welfare have boyfriends. There's a certain ethical code here which implies that these relationships don't mean promiscuity and that the relationships are not unacceptable to the community. While these living arrangements are not ideal or what the women really want, it's a way of managing. These women are basically people who underneath have a great deal of respect for their lives, but in many ways can't show it except when it comes to taking responsibility for their own children and families and the concern they show for other people. I suppose they need the kind of encouragement we give them—that they are worthwhile.

The teenagers' attitudes stem, in part, from the fact that they see no real future for themselves. One's past experience determines what one's going to be doing, but even more, one's concept of what the future holds can determine one's present activity. I think it's within the last couple of years that black people see a future for their kids if they get an education, whereas before it didn't help. One woman here has three aunts with college degrees from small colleges in the South, and they're all doing day work. But they know now that if their sons and daughters can go to college, or even to a high school with a technical training, that there is a future for them.

And then they will move out. There's no future staying within the project, not until the crime is brought under control, and there's a sense that the project is a place where good people live. Now for so many good people it seems to be a place only for bad people. In the old days when ward politics ran East City, even a poor person could get to his politician and get a hearing. The housing projects then were the places people lived in if they knew a politician. They had a status, they were citizens, they were voters, and their local politicians wrote them a letter. They got in because they knew someone important. They had a different self-concept then than they do now. Today entry into this housing system is through a social agency because you have problems related to poverty. The project may house the same kind of people, but their perception of themselves is different. My perception of myself has changed, too, since I came to live here.

When we first moved in I went to cash a check in the supermarket. I showed my driver's license and asked for a courtesy card. The man in the booth had no idea who I was. He wasn't being fresh but kind of condescending, and he said, "Oh Pattie, Babe, we don't give courtesy cards here. This is only welfare and factory people."

Groups? Yes, there are certain informal groups in the project. For instance, we have gotten to know most of the families in our building, so we can count on them in an emergency and they can count on us. The mothers aren't particularly friendly with each other, but they don't fight, and their kids get along. In general, there's not much of a sense of community, and the usual kinds of organizations that would promote a sense of community in a neighborhood don't exist in Bracken Field. The schools, which are natural places for mothers to meet and know each other, are divorced from the community. The churches, of course, should be the best meeting grounds for people to share a sense of community, but the church (the one place in which all are equal, regardless of background, income or education) is not active. The supermarket is the only place that is a common gathering ground for people, and it's not a very good one.

The overall impression is that nobody really cares about the poor in this country. It's not just the poor with families. We've had contact with the elderly, who are mostly white Irish, living on their pensions, very proud people. They live in the housing project mostly because their rent is only forty-five dollars a month, and they're too proud to want to be dependent on others. They're either people who have no relatives, or their sons and daughters are not bothering with them. Of course, they have the same problems with the police and with the community that they really are not a part of. And nobody really cares. The elderly are no longer productive, no longer a vital part of society and cut off from their own families as well. Because these old people have no family, they are put into buildings for the elderly, in areas of poverty and high crime, where they are the ones least capable of defending themselves. It just doesn't make sense. The only sense it makes is that if society really cared they could and would do it differently.

I was brought up in the Mid-West, and I used to think that beauty of surroundings was very important. I no longer emphasize the importance of nature, it's really the people that make the difference. There are areas in the suburbs with beautiful surroundings where the people are so sterile, so self-satisfied, and so narrow in their outlook that it's almost stifling.

I think the service of the Health Center is very much appreciated. In East City, with the lack of public transportation, the convenience of the Center is very important. It's important for the kids, and also for the women who can come to the center for prenatal care and not have to wait at the hospitals. Because of the particular area they live in, they've seen very little concrete services from other organizations. At least the Health Center is doing what it says it should be doing, it's giving health care.

I think, of course, the major problems are not health. When there's been criticism of the Center, it's that the Center has perhaps not recognized problems realistically. I think the residents do want to see some sort of advocacy role for the Health Center, from the health point of view. For instance, they want the Center to agitate for police protection, better housing, better maintenance, extermination of rats, more recreational facilities, establishment of infant day care centers, centers for mentally retarded children, centers to treat drug addicts, and so on.

What strikes me when outside people come into the housing project for the first time is how they say, "Why don't you do something? If you'd all get organized, something could be done." They are not being realistic. After living here, you realize how complicated the situation is, and how complicated the political situation is in East City. In order that the residents become organized in the housing project, they must have more of the power that's necessary. I think the tenants turn a deaf ear and maybe for good reason. Maybe they are more realistic about their own situation than the white liberals who aren't able to change their own suburban town but feel the tenants can change their area.

Our neighborhood aides', our community workers', best assets are that they can really educate the professionals to reorient their conceptions of their own roles— to learn what is acceptable professional behavior and what is not. When families have multi-problems, and every agency has been called in and then given up, it's not fair for professionals to decide that a community worker can do something. For instance, there has been criticism that we have overinvolved ourselves with certain families of which the community says, "The only thing you can do with these families is just learn to live with them." If we spend too much time with families that just manipulate the agency, we miss opportunities to extend ourselves to others who could use our services with more benefit. If you allow yourself to be used, the community doesn't respect you.

To have some impact on the community is a full time job, particularly when the community is not organized; so it's unfair to expect a Health Advisory Group to educate the whole community in terms of health. This group has played a very important role in protecting the Health Center from criticism from other community agencies. They handle other community leaders much better than you and I could. They've also defended the role of the professionals to other agencies in a period when there's been a great deal of antiprofessional or anti-hero kind of sentiment. That's been an important function.

We can't be naive about this neighborhood. It's like any other neighborhood with vested interests and corruption. Even neighborhood groups and anti-poverty groups may not function any differently from any other political system.

You ask my opinion on the possibility of community control of our Health Center? I'm not convinced that this is possible, not because of the people themselves particularly, but because we don't know who really controls what's going on in the country. It may be a cop-out to make a Policy Board of community people and tell them, "Now you control your Health Center." Federal funding depends so much on political situations which these people don't have access to. So much of control is intangible. On paper it may look like community control, but in reality so much depends on who knows who. We might be doing the community a disservice because we aren't steering them in the right direction for control. Somehow you have to get into the political system and have an input there.

Perhaps this is the role the Health Center should take in terms of the community. The Center should be very explicit about where it gets its funds, not just what the newspapers report. The Center should let the community know what the real medical politics of East City and Washington are, and what really makes the difference and how, if at all, the situation can be affected. I think this is something that students have learned in terms of their peace protests. They've learned that you have to elect people who are going to vote the way you want them to vote because these are the people who are going to vote for the funding.

You ask what I can accomplish by living in the housing project? I suppose in terms of the religious or human dimension, it may take three or four years before we really know what we can specifically accomplish or whether just the fact that we are living here has had some value in itself. Certainly, it has had value for us, not in terms of solving the poverty situation, but in terms of understanding how other people cope with the situation.

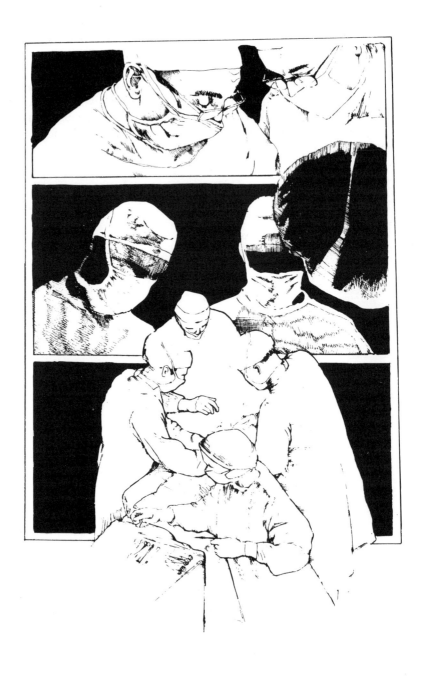

Chapter VI

Epilogue—Self—Interview

Self-Interview

Eva Salber, born and raised in Cape Town, South Africa, married a medical school class-mate and has four children. Interested as she was in her patients as people rather than in the illnesses from which they suffered, her focus was always the patient in relation to family and community. In regard to time, her professional life has been almost equally divided between South Africa and the United States.

A successful collaboration between patient and doctor requires mutual understanding. Health professionals customarily interview patients and present their case histories at "grand rounds," or "case conferences," but the process is seldom reversed. The interviews which make up the body of this book add to our understanding of the patients we dealt with. It seemed only fair to subject myself to the same procedure, and the idea of presenting my own interview, conducted by someone else occurred to me. In the end I decided to write my own story, since the substance of this book is the result of my interaction with twenty-one people and I did not want to introduce an outsider. And precisely because of this interaction I felt it necessary to reveal something of myself.

I was born and educated in South Africa, am married to a doctor and have four children. My interest in medicine has always been in the people who become ill rather than in the diseases they contract, and I have always believed that everyone should have access to medical care without regard to an ability to pay.

Two periods of my life, twenty years apart, highlight the direction of my career. The first began in Durban, South Africa in 1946 and ended in 1954; the second began in East City in the United States in 1967 and ended in 1969. At both times I realized sharply the helplessness and inability of a poor community to influence policy decisions affecting its life, but in 1967 I was better able to foster a movement towards consumer participation in the governance of a local health service.

In 1946 my husband and I joined the staff of the Institute of Family and Community Health in Durban, South Africa as salaried employees of the Federal Health Services. The Institute trained doctors, nurses and health assistants, to set up and work in community health centers, four hundred of which, at that time, were planned as the basic units of care for a proposed South African Na-

tional Health Service. Staff of the Institute set up model demonstration health centers in Durban, an industrial city and
seaport, and in Pholela, a rural African area, which were used for
service, teaching and research at the Institute.

Each health center which was established, as well as the demonstration centers, gave curative, promotive and preventive
health care to a "target" geographically defined, population. The
work was carried out in teams of doctor, nurse and health assistant
to give comprehensive out-of-hospital care to all the families in the
area. The definition of health care was broad and included nutrition, psychological counselling, environmental sanitation and
health education.

My husband and I acted as family doctors to an African
township in one of the demonstration health centers, where we put
into practice many of the concepts of the Institute, the most basic
of which was the employment of indigenous staff, trained for their
new roles at the Institute. In a sense only the doctors were
foreigners, since the nurses and health assistants were drawn from
the same ethnic groups as the patients we served. Without the assistance of indigenous staff we could never have attained an understanding and acceptance of population groups whose way of life
was so different from that of the doctors who served them.

Closely linked with the basic concept of the importance of an
indigenous staff was our recognition and acceptance of tribal chief-
tain leadership, extended family relationships and supportive
networks which existed in the community to whom we gave care.
A sympathetic respect for our patients' beliefs in the magical
causation of disease, the powerful role in healing of the medicine
man, witch doctor, diviner, and herbalist, was an essential adjunct
to our own modern, medical training in bringing help to our patients, though whenever possible we tried tactfully to circumvent
harmful indigenous practices.

Our years with the health center in Durban were humbling
because we saw the limited role of medical care in changing the
social and economic conditions of our populations. But we were
gratified also, when our services did make a difference in the death
and sickness rates, challenged as we were by the existence of ap-
palling poverty and malnutrition, and the difficulty of working
within a political system which contributed to these conditions.

Though the health center movement in South Africa did not fit the political climate of the times and the Institute was dissolved in the late 1950's, the ideas were picked up in other countries, including the United States, where the first health center established by Tufts University in Boston followed closely the South African model. When government policies became increasingly restrictive, we left South Africa in 1956 to begin a new life in the United States. A university in the North East had offered my husband a job in a Department of Health Administration. Some months later I was offered a job in another department of that university, and for the next nine years, I was fully engaged in epidemiologic research.

While this research was intellectually stimulating, I missed the warmth, the broad spectrum, the absorption and the challenge of the South African experience. Research alone, without the opportunity to apply the results, satisfied my brain but not my heart. At the same time the many years divorced from actual medical practice made the possibility of a job in clinical work less likely. In any case, I was becoming increasingly unhappy with the overall philosophy of medical practice in the United States. It seemed to me to be geared more to the interests and needs of the practitioners than to the patients, to over-specialization and "curing" with too little emphasis on "caring." The role of the family in the causation of illness, the importance of job satisfaction, the individual's ability to fit into his community seemed to be almost totally ignored in favor of a one-to-one patient-doctor relationship focused on organic disease. I missed the holistic approach of our Institute in South Africa. It is true that I saw examples of superb medical care, but I also saw examples of shocking neglect, and there seemed little hope in the near future for the development of a national health policy that would address itself to a more equitable distribution of health care resources—towards the removal of barriers to the access of medical care for all people—though some federal programs were addressing this question to a limited extent in the 1960's.

At this time when I was seriously questioning my attitudes towards the entire field of medical practice in the United States, even to the extent of considering redirecting my skills and interests to the fields of sociology or anthropology, the university offered me the directorship of the proposed Bracken Field Health Center for which funding was being considered.

The Bracken Field period has been fully described in the introduction. It was a painful wrench to leave colleagues, staff and patients at Bracken Field as it had been equally painful to leave the health center in South Africa. Now, in North Carolina I have an academic appointment in a Department of Community Health Sciences.

I am not an academic by choice. Slowly, and rather cautiously this time, I am beginning to relate to another community. The pattern is familiar. We are in the midst of conducting a household survey . . . .

Acknowlegments

I wish to thank Dr. Paul Denson, Director of the Harvard Center for Community Health and Medical Care and Dr. E. Harvey Estes, Chairman of the Department of Community Health Sciences, Duke University Medical Center, both of whom at different times allowed me the use of office space and secretarial assistance while working on material for the book. I am grateful to the late Constance E. Smith and the Radcliffe Institute for a grant which enabled me to purchase the tape recorder and typewriter used in this study.

My friend Dr. Robert Morris, Professor, Florence Heller Graduate School for Advanced Studies in Social Welfare, Brandeis University, encouraged me to persist in my writing when others were lukewarm. Mrs. Lucy Wilson of New York City, a good friend, was invaluable in the role of editorial assistant.

Mrs. Anne Alach, my former secretary, spent countless hours transcribing the original tapes. Her personal loyalty and devotion to me over the years is beyond praise. I am fortunate, indeed, with her successor, Mrs. Georgia Hunter who typed several versions of the edited interviews as well as the final manuscript.

It is hard to single out only a few individuals who have been particularly helpful, since I have been singularly favored with warm and steadfast colleagues, but I must acknowledge a very special debt of gratitude to Mrs. Kathleen (Chou Chou) Crampton.

My friend and colleague, Dr. Jack Geiger, more than any other individual I know, understands the effect of poverty on health. He expresses in a few pages in the preface to this book what I have attempted to say in a whole book. I thank him most sincerely.

Some of the people I interviewed ask me from time to time how "our book" is getting along. It is indeed their book. Without them the book would not exist. They broadened my horizons and enriched my life. I am grateful for this opportunity to convey their thoughts and words to a wider audience.

Library of Congress Cataloging in Publication Data

Salber, Eva J
  Caring and curing.

  1. Community health services—United States—
Citizen participation. 2. Social medicine. I. Title.
[DNLM: 1. Community health services—United States.
2. Social medicine—United States. WA30 S161c]
RA418.S26   362.1'2'0973   74-34171
ISBN 0-88202-021-8